Biomaterials in Modern Medicine

The Groningen Perspective

Biomaterials in Modern Medicine

The Groningen Perspective

editors

Gerhard Rakhorst
Rutger Ploeg

University of Groningen, The Netherlands

World Scientific

NEW JERSEY · LONDON · SINGAPORE · BEIJING · SHANGHAI · HONG KONG · TAIPEI · CHENNAI

Published by

World Scientific Publishing Co. Pte. Ltd.

5 Toh Tuck Link, Singapore 596224

USA office: 27 Warren Street, Suite 401-402, Hackensack, NJ 07601

UK office: 57 Shelton Street, Covent Garden, London WC2H 9HE

Library of Congress Cataloging-in-Publication Data
Biomaterials in modern medicine : the Groningen perspective / editors, Gerhard
Rakhorst, Rutger Ploeg.
     p. ; cm.
    Includes bibliographical references and index.
    ISBN-13: 978-981-270-956-1 (hardcover : alk. paper)
    ISBN-10: 981-270-956-8 (hardcover : alk. paper)
   1. Biomedical materials. 2. Prosthesis--Design. 3. Medical devices--Design and construction.
  I. Rakhorst, G. II. Ploeg, Rutger Jan, 1954-
   [DNLM: 1. Biocompatible Materials. 2. Prosthesis Design--methods. 3. Equipment Design--
methods. WE 172 B6143 2007]
  R857.M3B5727 2007
  610.284--dc22
                        2007038228

British Library Cataloguing-in-Publication Data
A catalogue record for this book is available from the British Library.

First published 2008 (Hardcover)
Reprinted 2016 (in paperback edition)
ISBN 978-981-3203-44-0

Typeset by Stallion Press
Email: enquiries@stallionpress.com

Contents

List of Contributors

Bulstra, S.K., MD, PhD
Department of Orthopedics
University Medical Center Groningen
Hanzeplein 1
9713 GZ Groningen
The Netherlands

Busscher, H.J., PhD
Department of BioMedical Engineering
University Medical Center Groningen
A. Deusinglaan 1
9713 AV Groningen
The Netherlands

Diercks, R.L., MD, PhD
Department of Orthopedics
University Medical Center Groningen
Hanzeplein 1
9713 GZ Groningen
The Netherlands

Engelsman, A.F., MD
Department of BioMedical Engineering
University Medical Center Groningen
A. Deusinglaan 1
9713 AV Groningen
The Netherlands

Erasmus, M.E., MD
Thorax Department
University Medical Center Groningen
Hanzeplein 1
9713 GZ Groningen
The Netherlands

Gu, Y.J., MD, PhD
Department of BioMedical Engineering
University Medical Center Groningen
A. Deusinglaan 1
9713 AV Groningen
The Netherlands

ten Hallers, E.J.O., MD, PhD
Department of Otorhinolaryngology and
    Head and Neck Surgery
University Medical Center St. Radboud
Geert-Grooteplein Zuid-10
6525 GA Nijmegen
The Netherlands

Herrmann, I.F., MD, PhD
Department of Otorhinolaryngology
European Hospital
Via Portuense 700
00149 Rome
Italy

van Horn, J.R., MD, PhD
Department of Orthopedics
University Medical Center Groningen
Groningen
The Netherlands
and
Wageningse Berg 104
3524 LS Utrecht
The Netherlands

van der Houwen E.B.
Department of BioMedical Engineering
University Medical Center Groningen
Groningen
A. Deusinglaan 1
9713 AV
The Netherlands

Hummel, J.M., PhD
Science Technology Health and Policy Studies School of
    Management and Governance University of Twente
Postbus 217
7500 AE Enschede
The Netherlands

Koopmans, S.A., MD, PhD
Department of Opthalmology
University Medical Center Groningen
Hanzeplein 1
9713 GZ Groningen
The Netherlands

van Kooten, T.G., PhD
Department of BioMedical Engineering
University Medical Center Groningen
A. Deusinglaan 1
9713 AV Groningen
The Netherlands

Kuijer, R., PhD
Department of BioMedical Engineering
University Medical Center Groningen
A. Deusinglaan 1
9713 AV Groningen
The Netherlands

van der Laan, B.F.A.M., MD, PhD
Department of Otorhinolaryngology
University Medical Center Groningen
Hanzeplein 1
9713 GZ Groningen
The Netherlands

Maathuis, P.G.M., MD, PhD
Department of Orthopedics
University Medical Center Groningen
Hanzeplein 1
9713 GZ Groningen
The Netherlands

Mahieu, H.F., MD, PhD
Department of Otorhinolaryngology
Vrije University Amsterdam
De Boelelaan 1117
1081 HV Amsterdam
The Netherlands

Meek, M.F., MD, PhD
Department of Plastic Surgery
University Medical Center Groningen
10 Fordyce Close Chellaston
Derby DE73 1YD
United Kingdom

van der Mei, H.C., PhD
Department of BioMedical Engineering
University Medical Center Groningen
A. Deusinglaan 1
9713 AV Groningen
The Netherlands

Neut, D., PhD
Department of BioMedical Engineering
University Medical Center Groningen
A. Deusinglaan 1
9713 AV Groningen
The Netherlands

Nicolai, J.P.A., MD, PhD
Department of Plastic Surgery
University Medical Center Groningen
Hanzeplein 1
9713 GZ Groningen
The Netherlands

van Oeveren, W., PhD
Department of BioMedical Engineering
University Medical Center Groningen
A. Deusinglaan 1
9713 AV Groningen
The Netherlands

Rakhorst, G., PhD
Department of BioMedical Engineering
University Medical Center Groningen
A. Deusinglaan 1
9713 AV Groningen
The Netherlands

Renardel de Lavalette, V.W., MD, PhD
Department of Opthalmology
University Medical Center Groningen
Hanzeplein 1
9713 GZ Groningen
The Netherlands

Schutte, H.K., MD, PhD
Department of BioMedical Engineering
University Medical Center Groningen
A. Deusinglaan 1
9713 AV Groningen
The Netherlands

Tack, J.W., PhD
Department of BioMedical Engineering
University Medical Center Groningen
Klipper 24
9801 MT Zuidhorn
The Netherlands

Thuring, C.M.A., PhD, DVM
Animal Welfare Officer
Groningen University
A. Deusinglaan 50
9713 AZ Groningen
The Netherlands

Verkerke, G.J., PhD
Department of BioMedical Engineering
University Medical Center Groningen
A. Deusinglaan 1
9713 AV Groningen
The Netherlands

Chapter 1

Introduction

J.P.A. Nicolai* and G. Rakhorst†

In modern medicine, technology plays a prominent role in the diagnosis of diseases and treatment of patients. As a consequence, healthcare requires new generations of medical doctors and engineers: medical doctors who are familiar with the latest technical developments in their field, and engineers who have knowledge about the human body-anatomy, physiology, pathology, etc. Development of medical products requires a close cooperation between doctors and engineers. Product development is a multidisciplinary and time consuming activity. In this chapter, the artificial kidney and silicone breast implants are described from a historical perspective to emphasize the long development times of medical devices. A list of medical grade materials is enclosed in the Appendix of this book.

The student should be able to explain why BioMedical Engineering is a multidisciplinary research area by its definition, and should understand the meaning of an innovation, a biomaterial and the role of medical doctors and engineers in medical product development.

*Department of Plastic Surgery, University Medical Center Groningen, Hanzeplein 1, 9713 GZ Groningen, The Netherlands.
†Department of BioMedical Engineering, University Medical Center Groningen, A. Deusinglaan 1, 9713 AV Groningen, The Netherlands.

1

Introduction

Biomedical engineering (BME) is an multidisciplinary field that spans interdisciplinary boundaries and connects the engineering and physical sciences to the biological sciences and medicine in a multi-disciplinary setting, to develop or apply new technologies in patient-oriented research and clinical healthcare. The scope of this rather young field of science covers many different medical applications, varying from the development and application of new medical imaging techniques (MRI, PET, X-ray scanning, etc.) and biochemical test kits for the assessment of organ function, cell function, cell-material interactions, blood-material interactions, to the development of medical devices like orthopedic implants, blood purification devices, mechanical circulatory support systems, etc. In tissue engineering and regenerative medicine, engineering techniques are used to facilitate culturing of cells outside the body or for changing the behavior of cells.

Due to the multidisciplinarity of BME, optimal communication between medical and technical specialists is of utmost importance. It seems that medical doctors and engineers speak different languages: doctors use terms and definitions which are often based on Latin words, while engineers like to use chemical or mathematical formulas in their language. Examples of the different communication barriers that have to be overcome are schematically demonstrated in Fig. 1, in which the development of a medical device is schematically presented as a cycle of activities.

In order to develop a new device that can be applied clinically, extensive communication is required between the potential user (the clinician) and the developer (the engineer). Whenever the developer does not understand what the user needs, the chances are high that the developed product will never find its way to the medical market. In the idea phase, new concepts have to be generated and initial sketches must be transformed into technical drawings. In this phase, communication among the engineers of different backgrounds — biomechanics, materials science and electrical engineering — is needed to build a first prototype. Often, new test set-ups have to be developed and built to

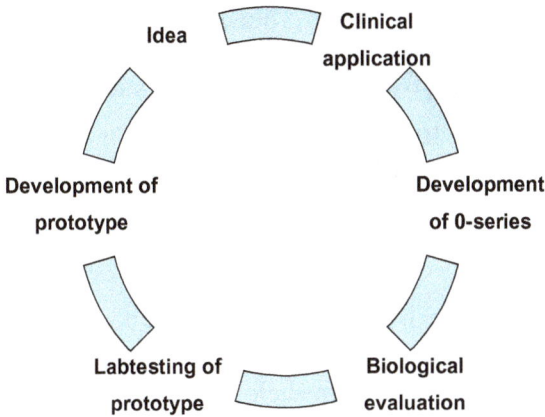

Fig. 1. Scheme of the different phases of the development of a medical device: from idea to clinical application. The curved blocks resemble the communication barriers that have to be overcome in order to realize the following product phase.

test prototypes on their functionality. Also, based on the potential risk of hazard, medical devices are classified into risk classes I, IIA, IIB and III. Depending on its contact with the skin or with other tissues or blood, and the duration of this contact, a number of biological tests (cell cultures and animal experiments) are required to prove the biological safety of the novel product. In the biological evaluation phase, communication between engineers, biologists, veterinary surgeons or clinicians is needed to define how these tests can best be performed and how the results should be interpreted. Once the technical requirements of the university prototype have been met, a small series production is needed to obtain a number of identical prototypes for animal studies. Generally, universities have to decide at this stage of development whether and when they want to transfer the developed technology to the industry. After technology transfer, the industry will have to develop its industrial prototypes, using its own manufacturing techniques to build a safe and affordable product. Furthermore, a clinical protocol has to be defined and must be evaluated by a medical ethics committee and national healthcare institutions for the purpose of obtaining permission for a first clinical application. For a clinical study, insurance has to be arranged, technical files have to be completed, and the study has to be documented and reviewed. Finally, when a new medical device has been applied clinically in a number of patients (phase-1 study), the industry can apply for CE certification or FDA approval and introduce the device on the medical market.

It does not need much imagination to understand that medical product development is a long lasting process. For example, it took more than 12 years of development time before the heart assisting blood pumps, like the Novacor® (developed at the Stanford University, USA) and the Pulse-Cath® (developed at the University of Groningen, The Netherlands) were introduced on the market. New pharmacological products need even more time before doctors can prescribe them to treat diseases. If one would like to develop a new device, using new non-medical grade materials, one may have to deal with the timespan that is needed to prove that the material is safe, as well as with the timespan to prove that the new application is safe. This is the reason why many chemical companies prefer to modify the surface characteristics of their produced materials with coatings, instead of developing new materials from scratch and have these certified for medical application. The long timespans needed before a product can be marketed pose a severe risk that once the device or medicine is introduced on the market, the technology used has become outdated already. In Fig. 2, the milestones in the development of the artificial kidney are listed. The timespan between the initial idea of using diffusion and osmosis by Thomas Graham (1861) for the detoxification of bodyfluids and the first clinical application of the artificial kidney by Willem Kolff (1946) was 85 years. The first device was introduced on the medical market 10 years later (Brigham-Kolff kidney). In the case of the artificial kidney, the clinical application depended strongly on the availability of bio-compatible materials (cellophane, cuprophane), machine techniques (rotating drum, coil technique) and new anticoagulants (heparin).

Reduction in the development time may be achieved by employing management techniques. With project management, the development of a product is divided into different tasks and timeframes in which certain activities are scheduled to take place, with the tasks each allotted a certain amount of money. When the different tasks can be performed at the same time, the so-called concurrent engineering method,

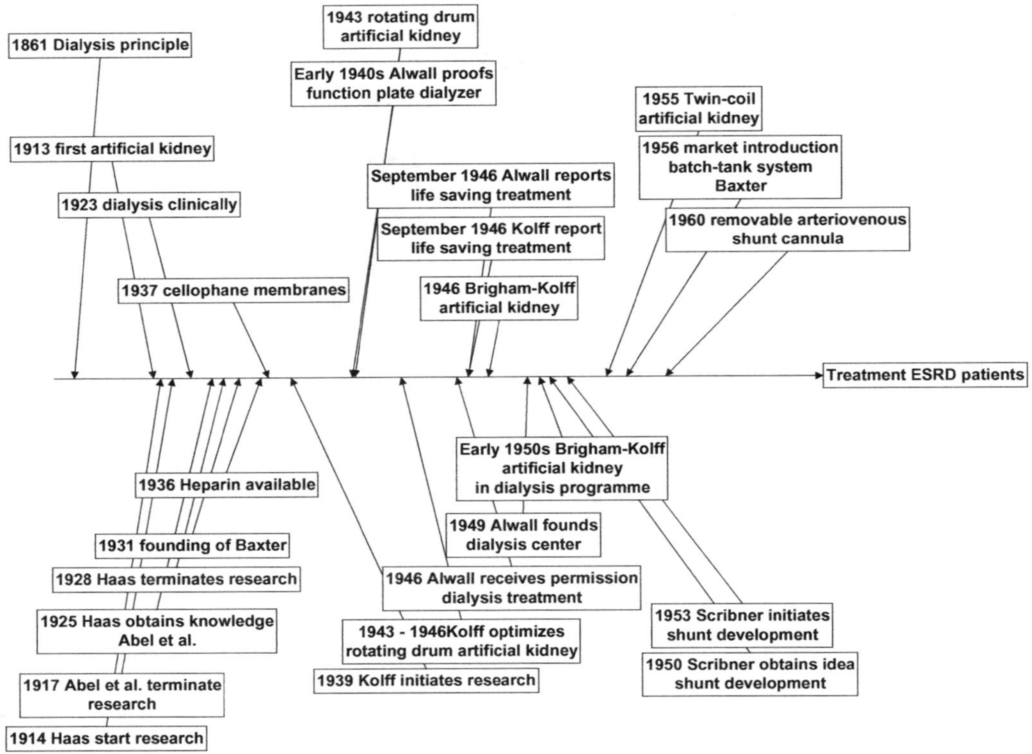

Fig. 2. Overview of the milestones in the development of the artificial kidney (Cijsouw *et al.*, 2005).

the development time will be much shorter than when all the tasks are performed in a linear manner. Knowledge management focuses on the availability of knowledge at the right moment, on the type of knowledge (sensory, tacit, coded) and on the transfer of knowledge from one project stage to the next. Medical technology assessment (MTA) aims at defining whether a new product performs better than an existing one, or whether the introduction of a new device results in a reduction of the costs of healthcare (cost-benefit studies).

> The fastest way to develop a medical device is to implement concurrent engineering techniques in the project management.

Biomedical research is performed at the frontiers of science. New products or techniques must be better than the existing ones; new ideas must be innovative and lead to innovations. Innovations can be based on copying an existing technique (imitative innovation); stepwise improvement of an existing technique (incremental innovation); or development of a totally new concept (radical innovation).

As mentioned before, medical devices are categorized according to the potential risk of harm they can induce on a human body in case of technical failure. Devices can either have no direct contact with the skin or other body tissues (e.g. X-ray machine), or have contact with the skin or other body parts. If there is contact, it can be a superficial contact like a bandage, a short contact with the blood stream (infusion bag), or a longtime contact with blood (heart assist device), bone tissue (bone implants) or other tissue (breast implant). Depending on the size (surface area), shape and physicochemical properties of the material, a body will activate blood cells of the immune system and/or coagulation system to protect itself against unwanted antigens. The inflammatory response may lead to rejection of an implant or blood clots may form on a blood contacting device. Some materials are more compatible with living cells than others. Materials that are suitable for contact with tissues or blood are called biomaterials. Non-resorbable biomaterials hardly induce inflammatory responses or clot formation and possess good biocompatibility properties. Resorbable biomaterials disappear from the body after mild inflammatory responses, generally through hydrolysis. Using advanced tissue engineering techniques, cultured living cells can be brought into a container where they can be kept alive and mimic certain organ functions. The first hybrid organ that has been developed and clinically applied is the bioartificial liver.

> Bioreactors should be developed by biologists and biomedical engineers: bridging tissue culturing techniques with mechanical engineering and fluid dynamics.

A biomaterial is any non-drug material that can be used to treat, enhance or replace any tissue, organ or function in an organism. In this respect, the materials used for a hand or leg prosthesis in the Middle Ages and even for George Washington's dentures were biomaterials. These, of course, were in contact with the skin or mucosa surface only. The materials, with which in certain cultures earlobes or lips are enhanced since time immemorial, are biomaterials. And these are in contact with the tissue under the skin surface, in fresh wounds. The same goes for the piercing of a nostril or a glans penis, age-old customs as well.

"Biomaterials" also refers to biologically-derived materials used for their structural rather than biological properties, e.g. collagen (a protein found in the skin, connective tissues and bone) as a cosmetic ingredient. Also, carbohydrates (biotechnologically modified) are being used as lubricants for biomedical applications and as bulking agents in the food industry. A list of contemporary biomaterials is presented in Table 1.

A medical device is any instrument, apparatus, appliance, material or other article, whether used alone or in combination, including

Table 1   A Non-Comprehensive List of Biomaterials used in (Plastic) Surgical Practice at Present and in the Past

POLYMERS – resorbable

Caprilactone/ glycolide 90/10	Panacryl
ε-Caprolactone	
Cellulose	
Ethylene oxide	with propylene oxide: "Pleuronic F-108," block polymer "DynaGraft" poloxamer
Glycolide 60% + dioxanone 14% + trimethylene carbonate 26%: Biosyn	
Glycolide + ε caprolacton	Monocryl
Hyaluronic acid ester	Hyaff
Poly(butylene-terephthalate)-co-(polyethyleneglycol)	Poly-active, Osteo-active
Polydioxanon	PDS (tensile strength 35 days 50%, 70 dg 0%; resorption 180–210 dg)
Polyethyleenoxyde	
Polyglactin	Vicryl (90% polyglycolic acid + 10% lactic acid), Polysorb (= vicryl + coating) (tensile strength Vicryl Rapide 5 days 50%, 12 days 0%; resorption 35–42 days; Vicryl Plus tensile strength 21 days 50%, 35 dg 0%; resorption 56–70 dg)
Poly-glecapron	Monocryl (colorless: tensile strength 7 days 50%, 28 dg 0%; resorption 90–120 day)
Polyglycolic acid	Dexon
Polyglyconate	Maxon
Polyglyceride	Trilucent
Polylactic acid	PLLA
Poly L-lactic acid (PLLA) 82% + polyglycolic acid (PGA) 18% copolymer: Lactosorb screws and plates	
Poly-L-lactide + poly-D-lactide + poly-glycolide: Delta system reorbable implants for osteosynthesis	
Polyvinylalcohol	Bioinblue, injectable

(*Continued*)

Table 1 (*Continued*)

Polysaccharide	hydrogel; soluble, but very slowly degradable
Propylene oxide	with ethylene oxide: "Pleuronic F-108," block polymer "DynaGraft" poloxamer

POLYMERS – non-resorbable

Acrylates – copolymer of 2-hydroxyethyl-methacrylate and ethylene-dimethacrylate: soft hydrogel contact lenses

2octyl-cyane-acrylate	Dermabond
Phenolformaldehyde	Canvesit
Polyacrylamide	Aquamid
Polyamide	nylon, e.g. Ethilon, Supramid
Poly-alkyl-imide	Bio-Alcamid
Polyaryletherketone	PAEK
Polycarbonate	
Polydimethylsiloxane	silicone
Polyester	Ethibond, Mersilene, Ticron, Surgidac
Polyester resins	
Polyetheramide	Ultem
Polyethylene	Medpor (porous, high density), e.g. chin implants
Polyethylene glycol	soluble, not degradable

Poly(glycol methacrylate) gel, armed with polyester knitted net: Hydron breast implants (1968)

Polymethylmetacrylate	PMMA, Sulfix
Polypropylene	Prolene, Surgipro, Marlex, Bard, Aptos
Polysulfon	
Polytetrafluoroethylene	PTFE, Goretex, Teflon
Poly-urethane	PU
Polyvinylalcohol	soluble, but not degradable
Polyvinylpyrrolidone	soluble, but not degradable (MISTI (Gold) hydrogel-filled breast implants)

Trimethyleencarbonate

ANIMAL or HUMAN DERIVED MATERIALS

Bovine collagen	+ chondroitin-6-sulphate on a silicone rubber sheet is Integra; major component of Zyderm, Zyplast
Calf bone	

DMB (Demineralized Human Bone Matrix) – Dynagraft: putty 64% DBM, gel 37% in reverse phase poloxamer medium

(*Continued*)

Table 1 (*Continued*)

Dura mater	
Isolagen	cultured autologous fibroblasts
Human fascia	
Hyaluronic acid	
Ox fascia	
Porcine collagen	Evolence 30

BONE REPLACEMENT

Calcium oxide, bioglass particulates of silicon, phosphorous oxide	NovaBone
Hydroxy-apatite tetra-tri-calcium phosphate	Mimix
Tricalciumphosphate + hyaluronic acid	Chronos-inject
37% Poloxamer gel medium + 64% D(emineralized human) M(atrix) B(one)	Dynagraft
Poly(butylene-terephthalate)-co-(polyethyleneglycol)	Poly-active, Osteo-Active

CERAMICS

Alumina
Carbon
Glass
Materials based on yttria-stabilized tetragonal zirconia

HYDROGELS

co-polymer of methyl-methacrylate and vinyl-pyrrolidone (osmotically active)	Osmed
Polysaccharide	

METALS

Aluminium (in alloys)
Cobalt-chromium-molybdenum
Nickel (in alloys)
Nickel-titanium (memory-metal)
Niobium (in alloys)

(*Continued*)

Table 1 (*Continued*)

Stainless steel	
Tantalum (also unalloyed)	
Titanium	coating for silicone breast implants introduced 2002, production terminated end of 2004
Tungsten (in alloys)	
Vanadium (in alloys)	

RESINS

(resins are polymers in
    cement form, e.g.:)
Acrylic (cements)
Poly(L-lactide) resins

INJECTABLES - resorbable

chitin	
chondroitin sulphate	
collagen	Zyderm I, Zyderm II, Zyplast, Resoplast (animal-derived collagen), Evolence 30
dermis	acellular human donor skin, Alloderm
gelatine	
glycosaminoglycan	Hyaluronan
human fascia	Fascian
hyaluronic acid	Acthyal, HAART, Hylaform (animal-derived (rooster combs) hyaluronic acid), Hyal-System (not cross-linked), Juvéderm (bacteria (Streptococcus Equi) derived hyaluronic acid, cross-linked by butanedioldiglycidyl ether (BDDE)), Perlane, Restylane, Reviderm (non-animal derived hyaluronic acid + dextran microspheres), Rofilan-Hylangel (non-animal derived hyaluronic acid (Hylan gel)), Touchline (not cross-linked)
polyglycolic acid	
polylactid acid	New Fill
poly(lactic-co-glycolic acid) microspheres	
polysaccharide	Hyaluronan (glycosaminoglycan), Hylan (cross-linked hyaluronan)

(*Continued*)

Table 1   (*Continued*)

polyurethane	
polyvinylpyrrolidone	as carrier in Bioplastique
polyvinyl-alcohol	Bioinblue (6% in 94% non-pyrogenic water)
tetra-methylene-diamine	

INJECTABLES – non-resorbable

acrylamide	Reonal
dermal collagen	porcine: Permacol
carboxymethylcellulose	CMC, carrier for hydroxylapatite microspheres, Radiance
cellulose	
collagen	Artecoll (PMMA microspheres in collagen)
hyaluronic acid	Dermalive (hyaluronic acid + hydrogel-acrylate particles), Puragen
hydroxyapatite	
methacrylamide	
methacrylate	Dermalive, Metrex
methylene-bis-acrylamide	
polyacrylamide	Amazingel, Formacryl, Argiform, Aquamid (2.5% cross-linked in water), Biogel (polyacrylamide hydrogel — the monomere is teratogenic)
poly-alkyl-imide	Bio-Alcamid
poly-dimethylsiloxane (silicone)	Bioplastique
(porous) polyethylene	Medpor
poly(methylmethacrylate)	PMMA, HEMA (2-hydroxyethyl-methacrylate (1936)); Artecoll (PMMA microspheres in collagen), Arteplast (same)
poly(tetrafluoroethylene)	PTFE, teflon paste, Goretex
polivinylalcohol	Bioinblue
polivinylpyrrolidone	in Bioplastique as carrier of silicone particles

INJECTABLES – by name

Acthyal	hyaluronic acid
Alloderm	acellular dermis of human donor skin
Amazingel	polyacrylamide
Aquamid	2.5% cross-linked polyacrylamide in water
Argiform	polyacrylamide

(*Continued*)

Table 1 (*Continued*)

Artecoll (1991)	PMMA (polymethylmethacrylate) particles (40 μm) in 3.5% bovine atelocollagen + 0.3% lidocaine HCl. (PMMA was patented in 1928)
Arteplast (19..)	is Artecoll, but with smaller PMMA microspheres (20–40 μm)
Bio-Alcamid	4% reticulate polymer of alkyl-imide in water
Biogel	polyacrylamide hydrogel
Bioinblue	8% polyvinyl-alcohol in 92% non-pyrogenic water
Bioplastique (1992)	silicone (polydimethylsiloxane) particles (100–600 μm) suspended in polyvinylpyrrolidone ("plasdone") carrier
Dermalive	40% hydroxy-ethyl-methacrylate, ethylmethacrylate in 60% hyaluronic acid
Evolence 30	atelopeptide porcine type I collagen, ribose induced cross-linking
Fascian	human fascia
Fibrel (1990)	porcine collagen + patient's plasma + ε-aminocaproic acid
Formacryl	polyacrylamide; replaced by Argiform
Goretex (1991)	expanded PTFE (polytetrafluoroethylene)
Hyal-System	hyaluronic acid
Hyaluronan	unsulphated glycosaminoglycan, a polysaccharide
Hylaform	hyaluronic acid
Hylan	cross-linked molecules of hyaluronan
Isolagen	cultured autologous fibroblasts
Juvéderm	hyaluronic acid
Juvelift	hyaluronic acid
Medpor	polyethylene
Metrex	acrylate and methacrylate spheres
Natucoll 3.5% (199..)	3.5% bovine atelocollagen + 0.3% lidocaine HCl
Natucoll 6.5% (199..)	6.5% bovine atelocollagen + 0.3% lidocaine HCl
New Fill	polylactid acid
Perlane	hyaluronic acid
Permacol	60% milled porcine dermal collagen matrix suspension in saline

(*Continued*)

Table 1   (*Continued*)

Puragen	hyaluronic acid, double cross-linking, + acrylate particles
Radiance	is Radiesse
Radiesse	is Bioform, smooth calcium-hydroxyapatite microspheres in aqueous polysaccharide (carboxymethylcellulose) gel
Reonal	acrylamide
Resoplast 3.5% (19..)	3.5% bovine atelocollagen + 0.3% lidocaine HCl
Resoplast 6.5% (19..)	6.5% bovine atelocollagen + 0.3% lidocaine HCl
Restylane (199..)	hyaluronic acid
Reviderm	hyaluronic acid
Rovilan-Hylangel	hyaluronic acid
Silicone, liquid (1955)	polydimethylsiloxane, 350 centistokes viscosity, withdrawn 1976
Touchline	hyaluronic acid
Zyderm I (1975, marketing approval 1981)	bovine collagen + 0.3% lidocaine HCl: 35 mg/ml
Zyderm II (1983)	bovine collagen + 0.3% lidocaine HCl: 65 mg/ml
Zyplast (1985)	bovine collagen cross-linked with glutaraldehyde + 0.3% lidocaine HCl

Injectables are classified as "Medical Devices with the addition of an active medical substance."

Breast implant FILLER MATERIALS

- Dextran
- Methylcellulose-hydrogel   Monobloc, Laboratoire Arion (with methylene blue)
- Polyacrylamide   Kiev, Italy
- Polysaccharide-hydrogel
- Polyvinylpyrrolidone   Misty Gold, Novagold
- Povidone-iodine
- Saline, serum physiologique
- Seaweed
- Silicone gel   McGhan, Mentor, Polytech-Silimed, Nagor, Eurosilicone, PIP, LPI, CUI, Lab. Sebbin, Lab. Arion
- Triglyceride (Trilucent)   Lipomatrix

the software necessary for its proper application, intended by the manufacturer to be used for human beings for the purpose of:

- diagnosis, prevention, monitoring, treatment or alleviation of disease
- diagnosis, monitoring, treatment, alleviation of or compensation for an injury or handicap
- investigation, replacement or modification of the anatomy or of a physiological process
- control of conception

and which does not achieve its principal intended action in or on the human body by pharmacological, immunological or metabolic means but which may be assisted in its function by such means.

According to ISP 14630, an implantable device is a device intended to be totally introduced into the human body or to replace an epithelial surface or the surface of the eye via surgical intervention which is intended to remain in place after the procedure. A medical device intended to be partially introduced into the human body through surgical intervention and intended to remain in place after the procedure for at least 30 days is also considered an implantable device. This application of biomaterial is not new either. In the 17th century, the subcutaneous implantation of mother-of-pearl or jade beads into the foreskin was described,[2] a practice remarkable enough for having succeeded at all at a time before the advent of asepsis and antibiotics. Piercings, therefore, are partially implanted devices and those penile implants totally implanted devices.

The practice of surgery has mainly been concerned with amputation, including the removal of tumors, for many centuries. Surgery then developed to include reconstructions and–in the latter part of the 19th century- to include transplantation surgery. Surgery has now entered a new phase—inductive surgery, i.e. the use of tissue engineering to induce the body to form a necessary replacement or desired enhancement.

Biomaterials have always been employed by surgeons. One has only to think of naturally present materials for suturing. Horsetail hairs, for instance, were still used for that purpose in the last decade of the 20th century in Eastern Europe. The introduction of biomaterials on a large scale only occurred with the advent of reconstruction, the surgical replacement of tissue. This was and is still done with transplants and implants.

How research and development of an implant evolves over the years can be well described, taking silicone breast implants (SBIs) as an example:

1930s The polymer poly(dimethylsiloxane) was discovered; under the name silicone, it is an invention in search of an application.

1962 Gerow en Cronin (USA) manufactured an envelope or shell of silicone (silastic) with a semi-fluid or gel-like silicone content.

1964 Arion (France) developed saline-filled breast implants with a silicone shell. Implants have a smooth surface and Dacron patches for fixation inside the pocket into which they are inserted.

1975 Fixation patches discontinued.

1976 Double lumen implants with saline in the outer lumen to diminish diffusion or migration of small chain polymers through the shell, which caused constriction of the surrounding tissue scar.

1979 Eight companies worldwide manufactured and marketed SBIs. Companies were sold and bought by one another and by others.

1979 Thicker shells were manufactured to prevent gel diffusion.

1985 A reverse double lumen SBI was marketed; it had an inner chamber which could be filled with saline to the desired volume; it also had the advantage of slowing down gel diffusion.

1987 Silicone-gel filled SBIs with a textured surface instead of a smooth one, appeared on the market; tissue ingrowth into the surface diminished the occurrence of scar constriction.

1989 Saline-filled SBIs with textured surfaces were marketed.

1993 Highly cohesive gel-filled SBIs were manufactured; the semi-solid gel contained few short polymer chains and showed virtually no diffusion of silicone.

1994 Pear- or teardrop-shaped SBIs were marketed instead of the round ones.

1995 Triglyceride as an SBI-filler instead of silicone gel or saline was marketed. X-rays necessary for mammography could penetrate the implant and can show up cancer, in contrast to silicone gel or saline which blocked X-rays, making multiple radiographies necessary for examination; the manufacture of triglyceride-filled implants was ceased within a few years because of saponification by body fluids diffusing into the implants.

1996 Hydrogel (polysaccharide, cellulose) introduced as an SBI-filler, but not allowed in every country.

2000 There were still no more than 10 SBI manufacturers in the world.

The manufacturing process of any device involves a cycle: basic research-design-testing-manufacturing-marketing-application-follow-up clinical and basic research, etc. (Fig. 1). The cycle leads to a spiral of ever increasing quality of the product. One sees that this is explicitly true for SBIs.

It is interesting to observe that the increasing interest of health authorities parallel the R&D of SBIs.

1991 A USA manufacturer lost a multimillion dollar lawsuit because a patient blamed her rheumatoid arthritis on her SBIs.

1992 The US Food and Drug Administration (FDA) called for a voluntary moratorium on the sale of SBIs in January until "safety and efficacy" have been proven by the manufacturers.

Countries like Australia, Canada, France, Italy and Japan followed the FDA moratorium blindly. In the UK and The Netherlands, health authorities consulted the plastic surgeons and decided not to limit the sale of SBIs whatsoever. In April 1992 the FDA lifted the moratorium for cases of breast reconstruction after operation in cancer patients, but continues the ban for aesthetic purposes. The silicone-affaire is born.

1997   In Europe, France was the only country to continue to ban SBIs.
1998   The Europarliament receives petitions from "silicone-survivors" to ban SBIs in Europe. An impartial scientific panel in the USA reported that there is no evidence of auto-immune (or other) disease caused by SBIs.
1999   Similar reports appeared in the UK and The Netherlands, produced at the request of Health Ministries. The European Commission considered that SBIs are under the scope of Council Directive 93/42 EEC on Medical Devices (covering safety and CE-certification) of 1993; they confirmed that the liability of manufacturers was covered by Council Directive 85/374 EEC of 1985.
2000   UK issued an alert on hydrogel filled implants.
2001   France lifted the ban on SBIs. The Europarliament voted against a ban on SBIs and sent its decision to the Commission and the Council of Ministers. Member States of the EU were requested to have registries of patients and SBIs.
2005   The Dutch Ministry of Health had still not taken any steps to set up a database for registering patients and SBIs.

The profession, i.e. medical doctors are taking care of post marketing surveillance (PMS) for a large part.[4] PMS concerns:

(1) Reporting adverse events and side effects
(2) Retrieval and analysis of explants
(3) Tracing and tracking of patients and implants, for which registries are indispensable. In the case of SBIs, an international registry has been set up.[3]

In general, however, medical doctors receive little information on biomaterials during their training. They are readily accustomed to the suture materials and implants used by their teachers. When they are approached by distributors who want to introduce new materials, doctors are pretty credulous and only a few study the literature on the chemical composition of the new material. Nor do they ask which notified body issued a CE-mark. Many lend credence and confidence to the simple assertion "FDA-approved." As we all know, the FDA is more of a political body than an ISO and a CEN, which institutions heavily rely for scientific input. Take an injectible like Biogel, consisting of poly(acrylamide). It is virtually impossible to produce a 100% pure polymer and there will always be traces of the extremely toxic monomer, mono(acrylamide). Few doctors know this and even fewer question the purity of the materials as advertised by the distributors.

Hospitals have become conscious of this and do not allow its doctors to give patients medicines that have not passed through thorough screening by hospital officials. The same goes for implants. Thus, doctors are rendered help in scrutinizing new biomaterials and patients are protected from doctors implanting devices that they carry to the hospital in their pockets.

Despite all these precautionary measures, catastrophes still occur. In the case of the silicone-affair, examples are the triglyceride- and the dextran-filled breast implants. Both triglyceride and dextran are regularly given to patients intravenously and many believed that filling a breast implant with them, would be innocuous. The contrary appeared to be true. Dextran attracted water through the porous silicone implant shell and patients asked their surgeon a few weeks after the implantation when their breasts would stop growing. Triglyceride attracts proteins and other chemicals from the body fluids, resulting in saponification and production of oxygen radicals. Thousands of Trilucent (triglyceride-filled SBIs) have been implanted all over the world. It is now recommended that all triglyceride-filled breast implants be explanted.

> Medical doctors need to be educated in medical product development in order to understand device-related complications (infection, bioincompatibility, dislocation, etc.)

It was the reaction to the FDA's moratorium on silicone-gelfilled breast implants, that led people to not only look for other filling materials, but to make a profit by selling them, however experimental the material. The inadvertent vacuum caused by the unscientific (and rather political) FDA moratorium therefore caused many patients distress and worse.

In the case where a doctor is credulous, one cannot expect the patient to be distrustful or be suspicious of a new material. For example, even today male-to-female transsexuals have their hips enlarged with large amounts of fluid silicone injections, in which case the material slides through tissue planes all the way down to the ankle, causing painful swellings that are very difficult to treat, if at all.[1] There are still patients who have the girth of their penises enlarged with paraffin injections, resulting in granulomatous reactions that can only be removed by excision. Needless to say, the licences of the doctors performing such unethical practices should be suspended. Patients, on the other hand, need to be better informed, more critical and more aware of the danger of consulting "cowboys" in malafide private clinics with all the ensuing complications.

Doctors have become more critical and are increasingly involved in post-marketing surveillance: IQUAM[4] and IBIR[2] are proofs of that.

The near future will undoubtedly see tissue engineering (TE) blooming. The TE constructs consist of a scaffold of degradable biomaterials serving as a matrix on which autologous cells cultured for multiplication are sown. Growth factors may be added to increase the potential of the entire construct. On the one hand, TE will offer more possibilities for treating patients; on the other, they are expected to increasingly replace implants. The future is bright; the future is inductive surgery.

This book contains two parts. Part I describes the more fundamental aspects of biomaterials research, such as cell-material interactions, inflammatory responses, animal models for biomaterials research and technology assessment. Part II describes various clinical applications of biomaterials: a state-of-the-art, its limitations and an overview of the problems that still have to be solved. For each application, the anatomy and morphology of the location where the implant becomes positioned is briefly described.

References

1. Hofer SOP, Damen A, Nicolai JPA. (2000) Large volume liquid silicone injection in the upper thighs: a never ending story. *Eur J Plastic Surg* 23(4):241–4.
2. Teensma BN, Nicolai J-PA. (1991) Literaire filologische en moralistische bespiegelingen over de Siamese penisbel. *Bijdragen tot de Taal-, Land- en Volkenkunde (BKI)* 147(1):128–39.
3. www.ibir.org
4. www.iquam.org

Abbreviations

CE: Conformité Européenne
CEN: Comité Européen de Normalisation
FDA: Food and Drug Administration
ISO: International Standards Organisation
PMS: Post Marketing Surveillance
R&D: Research and Development
SBI: Silicone Breast Implants

Chapter 2

Design of Biomedical Products

G.J. Verkerke[*,†] *and E.B. van der Houwen*[†]

Biomedical product design involves a complex series of activities that has to be performed by a team which, in order to have sufficient expertise, must be composed of people of various disciplines. Design of biomedical products is quite different from designing consumer products. The main question is how to create high-quality biomedical products that can solve a medical problem.

A new design method has been developed for designing biomedical products, based on an iterative approach and characterized by five phases: an analysis phase, three synthesis phases and the use phase.

To enable medical, technical and industrial experts to work together, the fundamental differences between the three groups must be known and accepted. A second condition for a properly functioning design team is that are the required roles are filled. Finally, a character analysis of the team members can prevent or solve conflicts.

*Corresponding author.
†Department of BioMedical Engineering, University Medical Center Groningen, University of Groningen, A. Deusinglaan 1, 9713 AV Groningen, The Netherlands.

Introduction

In 1400 BC a toe prosthesis was found in Thebe, Egypt; it was made from wood and could replace a missing toe (see Fig. 1). Apparently, designing biomedical products is a very ancient science. During the Renaissance, much progress was made by scientists such as Michelangelo and Da Vinci, in studying the physiology of the human body. At this time scientists covered all scientific areas, making their approach truly multidisciplinary. Since then, science has become more and more specialized, and that, unfortunately, has prevented progress in biomedical technology. Only since the beginning of the 20th century has progress been made due to a renewed focus on multidisciplinary research. For example, Röntgen discovered X-rays in 1896 and Einthoven developed the ECG in 1903. Since then, many products have been designed, from hip prostheses and MRI-scanners to surgical robots and tissue engineering.

To have a good understanding of how to design biomedical products, the terms *design, biomedical* (technology) and *product* need to be defined first. Design is part of the innovation process. It starts with the formulation of goals and strategies and selection of new products, and ends with the evaluation of the use of a new product. Product development involves only the first part of this process

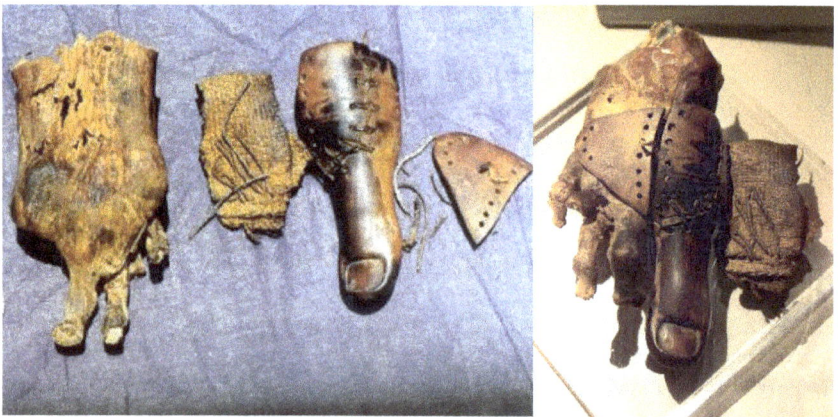

Fig. 1.   Toe prosthesis from Egypt (18th dynasty, 1424–1398 BC). Egyptian Museum, Cairo.

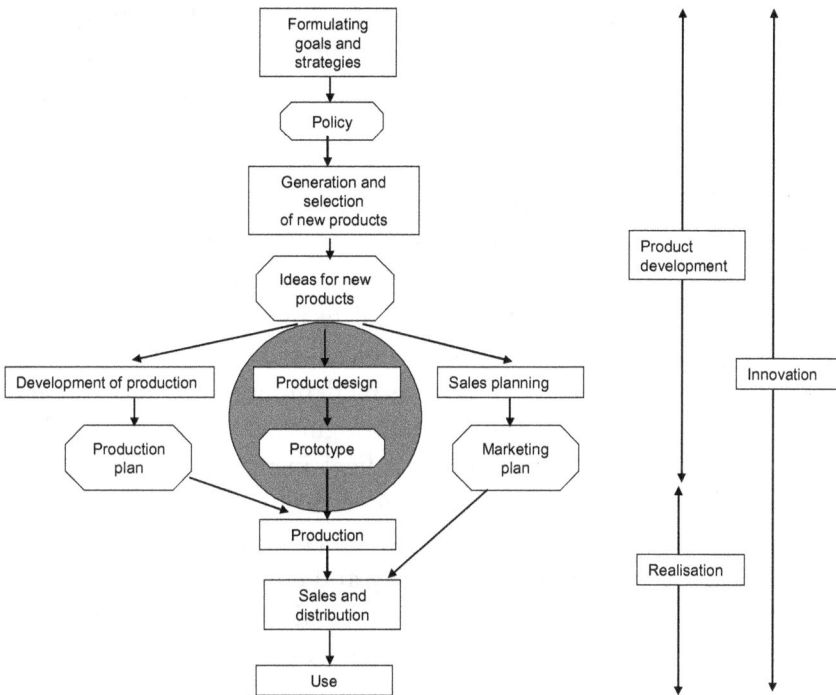

Fig. 2. The relation between design, development and innovation.[1]

and ends when a prototype is developed, including a manufacturing and sales plan. Design "only" involves the creative process that creates a prototype of a solution for a given problem (see Fig. 2). A product is a device or equipment used to analyze (diagnostics) or solve (therapy) medical problems.

Design of biomedical products is mostly performed by companies, but can also be performed by universities. Product design at universities is undertaken to realize new applications of existing knowledge, and is focused on the generation of entirely new products. Industrial product design is mostly performed to realize new applications of existing products and is, in general, focused on modification of existing products. Design at universities is, in general, not a core business, while research is. Design and research are essentially in contrast with each other, because research aims at creating new knowledge, while design aims at creating new applications of existing knowledge. For this reason both activities are very complimentary. Design requires generalists (people who know something of everything), while research requires specialists (people who know everything of something). Research is focused on analysis (analyzing structures to find their function and goal), while design is focused on synthesis (starting with a goal and function to find an appropriate structure).

To complete this definition section a definition of biomedical technology has to be given. Biomedical technology (BMT) involves the integration of engineering and medical sciences to improve diagnosis and therapy of patients. BMT is by definition multidisciplinary.

Three application areas can be distinguished within BMT: diagnostics, therapy and evaluation. Medical instrumentation, biosensors and medical imaging come under diagnostics; rehabilitation technology, prosthetics and orthotics, implants, and artificial organs under therapy; and clinical technology and ethics under evaluation.

To cover these application areas, several knowledge areas exist, such as biomechanics, transport phenomena, biomaterials, tissue engineering, medical physics, physiological modeling and interaction, medical informatics, artificial intelligence and biotechnology.

Methodical Design Process

A wealth of experience and many techniques and methods can be drawn on for designing consumer products. However, for designing *biomedical* products this expertise cannot be used directly, since the circumstances are quite different from designing consumer products. Therefore, a new design method has been developed for designing biomedical products. This method is based upon the method of Van den Kroonenberg,[2] Roozenburg and Eekels,[1] Eger *et al.*,[3] my 25 years of personal experience in designing biomedical products,[4–17] and the experience of my colleague E.B. van der Houwen. The essential aspects are:

- do things step by step for better focus
- archive your design process

- perform an extensive problem analysis
- abstract maximally to get an optimal range of ideas
- create many ideas, then the best idea could be one of them
- expand, freeze and select
- postpone decisions, and then you have more knowledge and thus can make better decisions.

The method is depicted in detail in Fig. 3. There are five phases: the analysis phase, three synthesis phases and the use-phase. Each phase contains several activities. All phases are characterized by an expansion phase, in which new aspects are created, a turning point, in which the situation is frozen, and a converging phase, in which the best aspects are selected. The nature of the aspect depends on the phase; in the analysis phase problems are inventoried and in the synthesis phases ideas and concepts are created. Another common

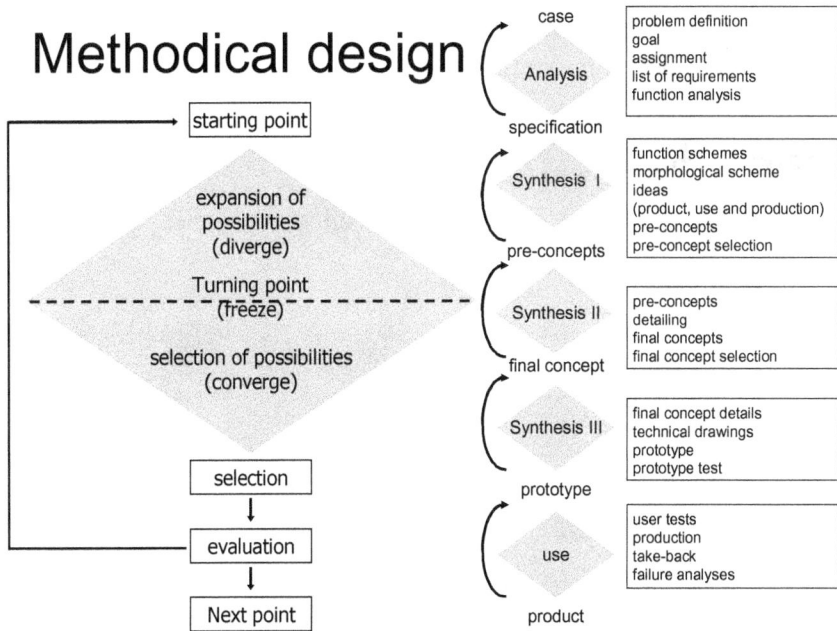

Fig. 3. Methodical process for designing biomedical products.

feature of all phases is that the end result of a phase is evaluated: Is the end result an appropriate answer to the starting point?

> Designing should be performed in a methodical and structured way.

Is it also still in line with the end result of earlier phases? This step is essential to ensure a high-quality final result, because it forces a check against earlier phases and prevents creating solutions for problems other than the one(s) proposed. Since with every phase more knowledge is created, this knowledge should be used to improve earlier results. This is actually a very annoying aspect of every design process: in the beginning there is plenty of design freedom, but limited knowledge, while at the end there is plenty of knowledge, but hardly any design freedom, since the final prototype is already realized and the manufacturing method is determined. This methodical process still differs not essentially from those, meant for the design process of consumer products. The essential differences show up especially in the analysis phase.

Analysis Phase

The analysis phase is composed of the following items:

- problem definition
- goal
- design assignment
- list of requirements
- function analysis.

Problem Definition

During the problem definition all people that are involved in the given problem are inventoried. An example: lower-back pain is an important cause of incapacity for work. Not only the person with lower-back pain is involved; so is his boss, his co-workers, his family and society in general. Another point of view is to realize that a biomedical product will be selected by the physician, financed by health insurance, bought by the hospital, used by the patient, and approved by the notified body, which is in contrast with consumer products, where all these people are the same.

In addition to the main problem, all those people will have related problems. To have a complete overview these problems have to be inventoried as well. For the given example this could result in the following overview:

- having lower-back pain for the rest of your life is a huge burden.
- to lighten the burden of the person suffering from lower-back pain, other people could facilitate his shifts, which aggravates their shifts in return.
- his boss has to achieve the same daily production, otherwise he will be fired.
- his family becomes depressed by his stories and his continuous bad mood.
- lower-back pain causes many people to be unable to work. This means high social insurance contributions, which is an economic problem for society.

A trap in formulating the problem definition is to formulate it as: "how to realize this solution?" After all, in many cases a physician will not tell you a problem to be solved, but a solution to be worked out. If this problem definition is used, the fundamental problem will not be traced and so only a single solution will be realized, which most probably is not the best one, or a solution for the wrong problem. Quantifying the problem is also difficult: how many patient suffer from this problem and how much do they suffer? (Pain is very subjective.)

Goal and Design Assignment

Subsequently, for each problem a *goal* can be formulated. Then for each goal, several design strategies (*design assignments*) can be created. Since there are many problems, there are even more design assignments that can be formulated. The expansion part of this phase is clearly present.

The converging phase is required to arrive at only one design assignment. That means a selection has to be made. Criteria that can be used are:

- price to create a solution
- time necessary to realize a solution
- feasibility
- chance of success
- the expertise that is available
- acceptance by the (many) people that are involved.

Another method of selection is to order problems causally. One problem is caused by another problem. So if the most fundamental problem is solved, most related problems are solved as well. However, it sometimes is not possible to solve the fundamental problem, because it is out of your control or insulated by laws, regulations or standards.

The design assignment that is selected largely determines the nature of the product that will be realized. The impact of available knowledge of the problem and feasibility of the design assignment, however, is minimal. So this crucial phase needs to be treated with due respect and attention.

If possible, two design assignments should be selected and worked out simultaneously. Also, frequent feedback (iteration) is necessary to decide if the feasibility of the other rejected design assignments is still worse.

List of Requirements

In a proper list of requirements all items are quantified. This makes it feasible to use the requirements as selection criteria for concepts that have been designed. Quantifying requirements for biomedical products is often very difficult, since no hard data are available. For instance, it is difficult to state how strong a device should be when you do not know the load that will act on it. So an estimation has to be made, which decreases the chance that the final product will be appropriate. For some requirements numerical simulation models can be used to make better estimations. Numerical tools exist that can calculate forces on body segments and bones for certain loading situations.

Function Analysis

Defining the function of a biomedical product is also a crucial phase, since it determines what the product must do. Defining its function depends mainly upon the body function that is lost or has to be supported. Since the human body is a very complex mechanism, several of its functions (such as walking and balance) and its part (organs) are not yet fully understood. This makes it difficult to design a product that resembles the body's functioning.

Use-Phase

The last phase of the methodical design process is the use-phase. In this phase the final tests will be performed, transfer to the industry is performed and series-production is started. Products that are used will be collected and analyzed for failures.

Tests

Biomedical products have to be tested extensively, especially where implants are concerned. Regulatory agencies (FDA in the US, CE in Europe) demand proof of the safety and functioning of products.

If the functional tests are successful, animal experiments have to be done to prove functionality in a living situation and to determine biocompatibility. Then a clinical trial will be performed, since all animal models have shortcomings when compared to the human situation. The clinical trial is followed by a multi-centre study to prove the concept in the hands of other physicians and to introduce the product in other hospitals. Finally a cost-effectiveness study will be performed to prove the economic value of the product.

Performing all these tests is both time- and money-consuming.[18] If in the end the product does not to function optimally (it has been found that in 50% of the cases the products appear not to fulfill all requirements at the end of the last test), a lot of time and money has been wasted and the use of that product will cause problems.[19] Regular feedback, as is integrated into the methodical design process and is proposed in the principles of Constructive Technology Assessment,[20] can prevent this outcome by changing the concept or prototype in time.

Transfer to the Industry

Products that are developed by universities often need to be transferred to industry. This phase is complex, since it will change the product from the prototype stage to a product that is produced in (large) quantities. This up-scaling is a major step that needs time and money and, of course, an industry that is willing to invest this amount of time and money. When industry can be interested from the start of the product's development, this step will be much easier than if an industry has to be convinced to take interest in this stage. Finding such an industry is difficult, since the products that are developed are meant for a selective, and thus small, patient group. The number of tests that have to be performed are numerous and a successful outcome is not guaranteed. Investing in such a product often is considered too risky.[1, 21]

Teamwork

Biomedical technology is a multidisciplinary field in which medical, technical and industrial experts work together, so cooperation between many people is necessary to realize a high-quality product.[22,23] Good cooperation should be very feasible, since all three groups

are oriented toward problem solving, have a rather technical background, and have a practical attitude.

Teamwork is not a trivial activity.

However, there are also a lot of differences between the three
groups that many people are not aware of. This ignorance often
frustrates cooperation and can even make it impossible.

Cultural Differences

Most differences are caused by a difference in culture and working
methods;[24,25] where culture is defined as a collection of ideas, norms,
values, behaviors and mutual understanding.

The cooperation between medical and technical experts, in particular, is more complicated than one would expect. When we char-
acterize both groups it can be seen that most characteristics stand
opposite each other (see Table 1).

Apart from different working habits and cultures, both groups
also have a different language. When one does not realize these differences, there is a danger of starting to dislike each other or, what
is even worse, find the other group inferior. Then any form of cooperation is impossible.

So how can these differences be dealt with? The most important
action is to acquire knowledge about each other's culture, working
methods, etc. Then this culture has to be accepted and respected as
a different but equal culture. For every step in the methodical design
process it must be anticipated how the other group will work it out.
If an approach different from one's own method is proposed, a compromise has to be found without violating the principles of the
methodical design process.

A good way to get to know each other's norms and values is to
compose the list of requirements together and to give a ranking to

Table 1.   Differences in Medical and Technical Culture

Medical Culture	Technical Culture
Organization is a hierarchy	Organization is a matrix
Decisions are made by an MD	Decisions are made by a group
Solution is for a single patient	Solution is for a group of patients
Technical procedures are followed	Creative procedures are used
Insulation from patients to mentally survive	Interaction with patients to analyze problem
Time for a solution is constrained	Solutions are extended for better results
Criticizing other MDs is not common	Mutual constructive criticism is common
Satisfied with global information	Only satisfied with detailed information
Solutions are found *ad hoc*	Solutions are well-considered
Aiming for proven, conservative solutions	Aiming for innovative solutions
Large solution database to select from	No solution database, to allow for maximal abstraction

the requirements with arguments. The arguments presented in favor of a specific ranking give particularly good insight into each other's norms and values. This method is known as the analytic hierarchy process and has been studied by J.M. Hummel[26] for application in biomedical product design.

Team Roles

A second condition for a properly functioning design team is to ensure that all team roles are present. Based on several studies, it is apparent that a team should be composed of people with different and complementary characteristics to achieve cooperation. Leary[27] developed, in 1957, a model with eight different character types. The Enneagram[28] defines nine different team roles: the perfectionist, the giver, the performer, the romantic, the observer, the loyal skeptic, the epicure, the protector and the mediator. Nowadays the Belbin model[29] is used regularly. Three categories are distinguished, each with three roles — an action, social and cognitive role. Only when all roles are present in a team can this team perform optimally.

Character Analysis

A third condition for an optimal design team is knowledge of the characters of the team members. After this analysis, potential conflicts can be foreseen and preventive measures can be taken. Also, conflicts can be handled better. The quadrant method is an efficient and effective tool for this analysis.[30] The basic feature of this method is that characters can be described in four categories — quality, thread, challenge and allergy — and that these categories are coupled (see Fig. 4). Performing one of your qualities too well will result in your thread. Improving your thread into the positive opposite defines your challenge. Performing your challenge too well defines your allergy, which in return is the negative opposite of your quality. Because all categories are coupled, by defining one character aspect you can add three other aspects of your character. This gives you insight into your character, and gives you the opportunity to improve it. After all, your thread is just an extreme form of a quality. And an allergy aspect of another person is only an extreme form of your own challenge.

Conflicts occur when the thread of a person resembles the allergy of someone else (see Fig. 5). By focusing on someone's quality instead of the extreme form of it, the thread, negative thoughts about

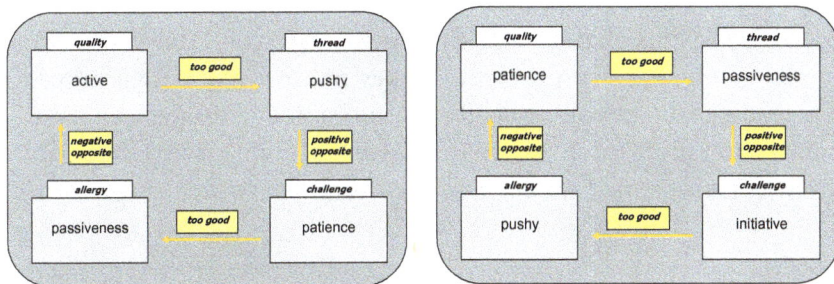

Fig. 4.   Examples of the quadrant method.

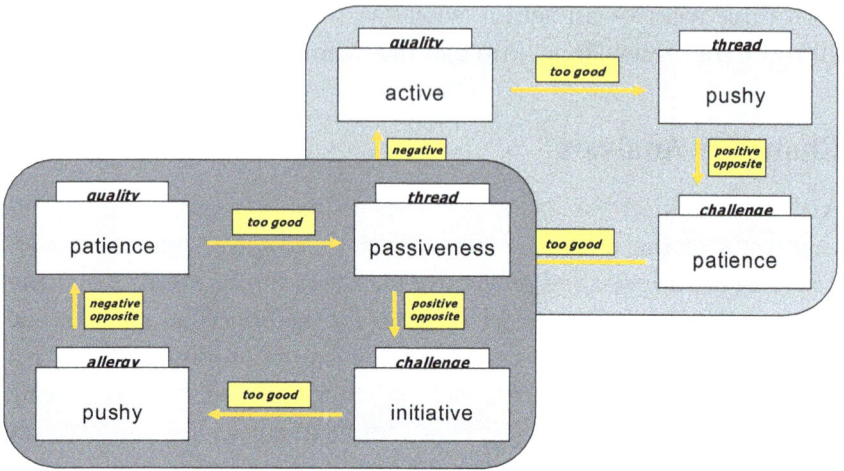

Fig. 5.   Application of the quadrant method for conflict analysis.

someone can be changed into positive ones, thus solving the conflict. And each conflict tells you a lot about your own character. Your allergy is, after all, an extreme form of your challenge!

Conclusions

The essential element in the design of biomedical products is a design team with sufficient expertise, thus with many disciplines. All team roles must be present. The team members must have knowledge of and respect for each other's culture. The methodical design process presented in this chapter is a structured way to perform all design stages. Analysis of the problem is a key phase in the design process. There are many problems, and even more design strategies (assignments). Iteration is an essential aspect, since with every step more knowledge is created that can be used to improve former phases.

Designing biomedical products differs substantially from designing consumer products.

With an optimal design team that cooperates respectfully and applies the methodical design method, it will be possible to create many innovative biomedical products that can contribute to improving the diagnosis and therapy of patients.

References

1. Roozenburg NFM, Eekels, J. (1998) *Productontwerpen Structuru en methoden* (Product design, structure and methods). Lemma, Utrecht.
2. Kroonenberg HH van den, Siers FJ. (1998) *Methodisch Ontwerpen: Ontwerpmethoden, Voorbeelden, Cases en Oefeningen*. (Methodical design: design methods, examples and exercises). Educatieve Partners Nederland, Houten.
3. Eger A, Bonnema M, Lutters E, Voort M van der. (2004) *Productontwerpen* (Product design). Lemma, Utrecht.
4. Geertsema AA, Boonstra CW, Schutte HK, Verkerke GJ. (1999) Design and test of a new tracheostoma valve based on inhalation. *Arch Otol Head Neck Surg* **125**:622–6.
5. Geertsema AA, Schutte HK, Rakhorst G, *et al.* (2001) A novel tracheal tissue connector for fixation of laryngeal prostheses. *Biomaterials* **22**:1571–78.
6. Loon JP van, Bont LGM de, Stegenga B, *et al.* (2002) Groningen temporomandibular joint prosthesis. Development and first clinical application. *Int J Oral Maxillofac Surg* **31**:44–52.
7. Mihaylov D, Verkerke GJ, Plaats A van der, *et al.* (2000) Design and test of the PUCA-2, a single valved left ventricular assist device. *Int J Artif Organs* **23**(10):697–702.
8. Polmans RPJ, Grootenboer HJ, Schraffordt Koops H, *et al.* (2001) Design and analysis of coupling methods for modular endoprosthetic systems as an alternative for the conical coupling. *Int J Art Org* **24**(5):304–10.
9. Verkerke GJ, Hof AL, Zijlstra W, *et al.* (2005) Determining the centre of pressure during walking and running using an instrumented treadmill. *J Biomech* **38**:1881–5.
10. Verkerke GJ, Lemmink KAPM, Slagers AJ, *et al.* (2003) Precision, comfort and mechanical performance of the Quadriso-tester, a quadriceps force measuring device. *Med Biol Eng Comput* **41**:283–9.
11. Verkerke GJ, Muinck ED de, Rakhorst G, Blanksma PK. (1993) The PUCA pump, a left ventricular assist device. *Artif Org* **17**(5):365–8.
12. Verkerke GJ, Rakhorst G. (2000) Design and test of an aortic access port. *Artif Org* **24**(5):395–9.
13. Verkerke GJ, Schraffordt Koops H, Veth RPH, *et al.* (1990) An extendable modular endoprosthetic system for bone tumor management in the leg. *J Biomed Eng* **12**:91–6.

14. Verkerke GJ, Schraffordt Koops H, Veth RPH, *et al.* (1989) Design of a load cell for the Wagner distractor. *Proc Instn Mech Engrs, Part H: J Eng in Med* 203:91–6.

15. Verkerke GJ, Schraffordt Koops H, Veth RPH, *et al.* (1989) Design of a lengthening element for a modular femur endoprosthetic system. *Proc Instn Mech Engrs, Part H: J Eng in Med* 203:97–102.

16. Verkerke GJ, Veenstra A, Schutte HK, *et al.* (1994) Design and test of a hands-free tracheostoma valve to improve the rehabilitation process after laryngectomy. *Int J Artif Org* 17:175–82.

17. Vries MP de, Plaats A van der, Torn M van der, *et al.* (2000) Design and in-vitro testing of a voice-producing element for laryngectomized patients. *Int J Artif Org* 23(7):462–72.

18. Hodgins D. (2004) Developing innovative implantable medical devices. *Med Dev Techn* 5:22–4.

19. Ward JR, Clarkson PJ. (2004) An analysis of medical device-relates errors: prevalence and possible solutions. *J Med Eng Techn* 28(1):2–21.

20. Hummel JM, Rossum W van, Verkerke GJ, Rakhorst G. (2000) Assessing medical technologies in development — A new paradigm of medical technology assessment. *Int J Techn Ass in Health Care* 16(4):1214–9.

21. McKay I. (2004) Novel approaches to innovation in medical device manufacture. *Med Dev Techn* 6:24–6.

22. Herstatt C, Hippel E von. (1992) From experience: developing new product concepts via the lead user method: a case study in a 'low-tech' field. *Journal of Product Innovation Management* 9:213–21.

23. Shaw B. (1998) Innovation and new product development in the UK medical equipment industry. *IJTM, Special Issue of Management of Technology in Health Care* 15:433–45.

24. NHS. *Culture – Professional and Managerial Cultures and their Impact on the Quality of Service.* (2000) Summary report of the key points emerging from the seminar discussion on Professional and Managerial Cultures, London.

25. Shelton JD. (2001) The provider perspective: human after all. *International Family Planning Perspectives* 27(3):152–61.

26. Hummel JM, Omta SWF, Rossum W van, *et al.* (1998) The analytic hierarchy process: an effective tool for a strategic decision of a multidisciplinary research centre. *Knowledge, Technology & Policy* 11-1/2:41–63.

27. Leary T. (1987) *Info Psychology.* New Falcon Publ, Tempe.

28. Palmer H, Brown PB. (1998) *The Enneagram Advantage: Putting the 9 Personality Types to Work in the Office.* Harmony Books, New York.

29. Belbin RM. (2004) *Management Teams: Why they Succeed or Fail.* Butterworth Heinemann, Oxford.

30. Ofman DD. (1994) *Bezieling en Kwaliteit in Organisaties* (Inspiraton and quality in organizations). Servire, Cothen.

Chapter 3

Animal Models in Biomaterials Research

G. Rakhorst,* *E.J.O. ten Hallers†* and
C.M.A. Thuring‡

For centuries animals have been used in medical research to obtain more insights into the functioning of the human body. Although animals differ from man, many physiologic processes are comparable and can be studied in more detail in animals than in man. In this regard animals are used for development and testing of new drugs, sera and vaccines, development and validation of new diagnostics, and development and training of surgical techniques under realistic (physiological) conditions. The need for animal experiments in medical research has come into question today. Animal welfare

*Department of BioMedical Engineering, University Medical Center Groningen, A. Deusinglaan 1, 9713 AV Groningen, The Netherlands.
†Department of Otorhinolaryngology and Head and Neck Surgery, University Medical Center St. Radboud, Geert-Grooteplein Zuid-10, 6525 GA Nijmegen, The Netherlands.
‡Animal Welfare Officer, Groningen University, A. Deusinglaan 50, 9713 AZ Groningen, The Netherlands.

groups raise questions such as, "Are we, as intelligent human beings, allowed to use and harm animals that cannot defend themselves?", and "Is it ethically acceptable to use animals for medical research while men and animals are so much different?" This chapter deals with animal models that are used in medical devices development and presents three case studies in which animals were used to mimic a clinical situation.

Introduction

In 2004, more than 600,000 animals were used in the Netherlands for animal experimentation purposes. Of these animals, 45% were used for development, production and control of sera and vaccines, while 47% were used for scientific research. Only 1.7% were used for education and training. In scientific research most animals were used in cancer and cardiovascular research or in research concerning other diseases (Registry Netherlands Food Safety Authorities, 2004).

Whether it is useful to perform so many experiments on living animals can be questioned. Animal species differ from each other and from man in metabolic activity, anatomy, morphology, the immune system and in behavior. Therefore, even when animal experiments have shown significant results, clinical studies are still needed to demonstrate that the studied phenomena exist in man as proposed. In other words, although animal studies may predict that some phenomena studied are equal to that in man, the real proof of principle still has to be performed on humans.

Russell initiated a movement to decrease the number animals used for research purposes, introducing the three Rs: Reduction, Refinement and Replacement (Russell and Burch, 1959, http://altweb. jhsph.edu/publications/humane_exp/chap4a.htm). Their way of thinking resulted in a more critical approach to animal experimentation by scientists and politicians, and has contributed to the establishment of national and European laws on experimental animals and animal welfare. Although societies in the Western world have become increasingly aware of animal rights, animal welfare and the need for reduction of animal experimentation, European and US legislation on medical devices (ISO 10993: Biological evaluation of Medical Devices FDA Guidance for pre-market notification submissions, etc.) demand that new medical products are extensively tested in animals on safety aspects, before they can be introduced onto the market and applied on a large clinical scale.

Replacement of animal experiments can be realized by using alternatives such as computer models, cell cultures, and physical models of circulatory systems (mock-circulations). Machine perfusion techniques and bioreactors using organs that are retrieved from slaughterhouses may reduce animal experiments in the near future as well. Sometimes the use of alternatives to animal experiments is more accurate than an animal experiment itself. For example, numerical models of the circulatory system allow us to calculate pressure or flow data at any place inside the body or in an organ, while these parameters can hardly be measured with conventional instrumentation techniques. Finally, appropriate use of biomedical data obtained from previous experiments performed by other researchers may prevent unnecessary use of animals in medical research as well.

> Computer models can calculate physiological data that cannot be measured *in vivo*.

This chapter emphasizes the need for refinement in animal experimentation: whenever it is decided that no alternatives are available to replace an animal experiment and it is clear that animal experiments are needed, these experiments should be performed under the best experimental conditions. In this way, technical failures are avoided and the number of experiments is limited. Some large animal models are described in more detail in this chapter to highlight the difficulties one might face in performing animal studies.

Animal Models

Definition: An animal model can be defined as an animal of which one or more specific characteristics (physiology, anatomy, pathology, etc.) mimics that of humans.

Animal Selection

In an animal model only a small number of specific characteristics, such as the size or shape of red blood cells, must be comparable with that of men. In most large animal models (dogs, swine, sheep, goats and calves) cardiovascular parameters like blood pressure, heart rate, blood volume, heart mass, etc. can be compared with that of humans. However, within the same group of animals, other parameters like gastric pH, electrolytes or glucose levels are not comparable because of differences in the metabolic and gastric system (ruminants, herbivores, omnivores, carnivores) of these animals and humans. In Table 1, hematological data of a number of frequently used experimental animals are listed to demonstrate species-specific normal blood values. In general, the choice of which animal species is best suited for an experimental study is based on both scientific and non-scientific arguments.
Scientific arguments include:

- Comparable anatomy or histology
- Comparable physiology
- Comparable pathology
- Comparable genes
- Comparable infectious patterns, etc.

Non-scientific reasons to use a specific animal species in a study include:

- Availability of the animal
- Costs
- Availability of suitable housing
- The researcher's experience with animal models

Table 1. Blood Values of Different Animal Species.[2-4] Averages or Ranges of Normal Blood Count Data in Various Animal Species. Notice that the Differentiation of White Blood Cells Differs almost between Each Species. Furthermore, the Size and the Amount of Red Blood Cells Vary over a Wide Range. The Same is True for the Different Platelet Numbers

	Unit	Mouse	Rat	Rabbit	Cat	Dog	Swine	Sheep	Cow
Hb	g/dl	10–16.5	11–19	10–15	8–15	12–18	10–16	8–16	8–15
HCt	%	39–49	36–54	30–50	25–45	30–55	32–50	24–45	24–48
MCV	fl	41–49	48–70	63	65–80	65–80	50–68	23–48	40–60
RBC	$10^6/mm^3$	9.20	6.5–9.5	6.5	5.5–10	5.5–8.0	7	9–15	5–6
WBC	$\times 10^3$	6–15	6–18	7–13	4–19	6–17	7–20	4–12	4–12
Differentiation									
Neutrophils	%	10–40	10–30	20–60	35–75	60–77	28–50	20–40	15–45
	$\times 10^3/mm^3$		1.7–3.4		2.5–12.5	3.6–11.5			
Lymphocytes	%	70	70	30–40	20–55	12–30	55	60	45–75
	$\times 10^3/mm^3$		4.8–12		1.5–7.0	1.0–4.8			
Eosinephiles	%	2–3	0.5	2	2–12	2–10	0.2	5	2–20
	$\times 10^3/mm^3$		0.03–0.08		0.0–1.5	0.01–1.25			
Monocytes	%	2	0.3	8.5	1–4	3–10	4	3	2–7
	$\times 10^3/mm^3$		0.01–0.04		0.0–0.85	0.15–1.35			
Basophils	%		0.00–0.03		0.0–0.3	0.0–0.3			
	$\times 10^3/mm^3$								
Platelets	$\times 10^3/mm^3$	160–410	150–460	125–270	300–700	200–900	100–500	100–800	50–750

- Availability of validated biochemical test kits (ELISA, etc.) that can be used in animals and humans
- The proposed animal model has been used by other scientists in the research field.

Van Zutphen *et al.*[1] describes in his handbook six steps to select an animal model.

Animal Handling and Transportation

Animal handling and animal housing have a great influence on the animals' well-being. Animals are not used to instrumentation or handling. Handling also differs from one animal species to the other. Monkeys are wild animals and, although some monkeys may get used to experimentation, most of them have to be sedated before they can be handled. For example, electrocardiographic examination of monkeys requires sedation to allow placement of the electrodes on the extremities or chest, and to keep the animal in a stable position during examination. On the other hand, personal experiences with electrocardiographic measurements in calves and dogs have demonstrated that when these animals were instrumentated for the first time, their heart rate went up to 180 beats per minute. However, heart rate hardly elevated during instrumentation when the animals were trained for a short time and became familiar with the handling. In this regard animal handling and proper training will influence the results of an experimental electrocardiographic study significantly. The importance of providing environmental enrichment and training animals on experimental procedures is generally accepted and has been included in the draft of revised guidelines on accommodation and care of laboratory animals of the Council of Europe (Convention ETS 123, http://conventions.coe.int/Treaty/en/TRaties/Html/123.htm. Moreover, publishing data of untrained animals might result in control data that differ from generally accepted baseline data (normal values).

> Animal handling and housing have a great impact on the behavior of experimental animals.

Besides the handling, the means of transportation (car, box, lorry) as well as the transportation conditions (use or non-use of sedatives) may result in stress, thus influencing all physiological parameters.

Animal Housing

Housing can be categorized in various ways. For behavioral studies animals are kept as much as possible within their natural environment. In behavioral studies fences are only used to prevent animals from leaving the territory of the institute or to limit their natural territory without influencing their natural behavior. Farm animals and laboratory animals are not kept in the open. They are housed together in stables or individually in cages. Some experiments need specific housing conditions. Specific Pathogen Free (SPF) animals must be housed under strict hygienic conditions. These conditions include that air that enters the cage is filtered, all equipment and food that is brought in is sterilized, and the animals used are obtained via hysterectomy to prevent that an animal can be infected during natural birth. In climate controlled rooms light intensity, light duration, day and night rhythm, humidity and temperature can be regulated from outside. Ottesen *et al.*,[12] listed the following conditions that animal housing should fulfill:

1) Mice, rats, guinea-pigs, rabbits and dogs must be able to have social contact with others from the same species
2) The animals should have enough freedom to move and need an enriched environment that allows species-specific behavior
3) The housing must allow individual animal species to fulfill their specific needs with regard to patterns of movement, control of

surroundings, security, safety, occupation, resting and eating patterns

4) The animal-human interaction should be considered.

In Table 2 the recommended space for commonly used farm animals is listed.[5]

Table 2.   Recommended Space for Housing of Large Animal Models

Animals/Enclosure	Weight, kg	Floor Area/Animal, ft² *
Sheep and Goats		
1	under 25	10.0
	up to 50	15.0
	over 50	20.0
2–5	under 25	8.5
	up to 50	12.5
	over 50	17.0
Over 5	under 25	7.5
	up to 50	11.3
	over 50[c]	15.0
Swine		
1	under 15	8.0
	up to 25	12.0
	up to 50	15.0
	up to 100	24.0
2–5	under 25	6.0
	up to 50	10.0
	up to 100	20.0
Over 5	under 25	6.0
	up to 50	9.0
	up to 100	18.0
Cattle		
1	under 75	24.0
	up to 200	48.0
2–5	under 75	20.0
	up to 200	40.0
Over 5	under 75	18.0
	up to 200	36.0

Note: *To convert square feet to square meters, multiply by 0.09.

Availability

Due to strict regulations by most national authorities, laboratory animals can only be obtained from registered farms or certified companies. All animals used are documented by their DEC number (given by the University Ethical Committee on Animal Experimentation), the experimental protocol and the invoice number of the company.

Practical guidelines for planning and performing animal experiments (checklist for Art. 9 officers):

- define the aim of the experiment and check whether an animal study is necessary (look for alternatives for finding the answers on the scientific question);
- seek multidisciplinary advice (from clinicians, technicians, animal welfare officers [Art. 14 Officers ex Wod] and biotechnicians);
- select an animal model and define the number of required animals to meet the statistical criteria to obtain significant results;
- prepare a working (or surgical) protocol including used anesthetics and surgical techniques, the use of analgetics and antibiotics, and discuss this with all personnel that will be involved in the study (biotechnicians, zootechnicians, researchers, etc.). Discuss housing, food, pre- and postoperative care, etc. as well;
- prepare a request for approval of the study by the University Ethical Committee on Animal Experimentation;
- after having obtained approval, make reservations for the use of the operating rooms, housing facilities, etc. and order the animals;
- after the animals have arrived check health condition and let animals acclimate to their new housing conditions for a period of at least seven days. Document the animals' welfare in a logbook, until the experiment has been terminated;
- prepare and check experimental set-up the day before the experiment will take place;
- perform the experiments and document all recordings.

Ethics

The way people think and care about animals is rather complex. For millennia animals have been bred and raised for food. In the food industry meat, milk and egg production are economic factors. The better farm animals are treated the better they grow and the more they produce. In this regard, prevention of infectious diseases has become very important. Not for the sake of the animals, but to prevent that a (temporary) decrease in production of dairy products might influence the economy.

On the other hand, for millennia animals have been kept by men as pets and have been treated with a focus on animal welfare, almost equal to humans. Pets are fed with high quality food, pets receive health examination and are vaccinated to prevent that they become ill. In this regard veterinary medicine and animal food industries can compete with human medicine and the human food industry in many ways.

The contradiction between eating animals and petting animals has influenced the way people think about animal experiments. Most people agree that some animal experimentation is necessary. However, most people also do not want these experiments to be performed on animals they are familiar with. Today society hardly accepts the use of dogs, cats, horses, monkeys and apes in animal studies, while pigs, sheep, goats, rats, mice, etc. seem to be better accepted by the public.

European and National Legislation

In 1986 the European Community published Directive 86/609/EEC, in which guidelines are set that are aimed at the protection of animals used for experimental and other scientific purposes. The Directive describes the minimal requirements that are needed to control the use of laboratory animals, and the minimum standards for housing and care. Furthermore, it describes requirements for the training of personnel handling animals and for researchers who are supervising the experiments. Although the Directive cannot be regarded as a European Law, it operates as a guideline for European countries, strengthens national laws, and acts as a standard on which new regulations on animal experiments can be established that contribute to a reduction of the number of animals used for experiments and the protection of animals rights and welfare.

In the Netherlands Law on Animal Experimentation (*Wet op de dierproeven*):

- article 2 describes the requirements for institutions to become licensed to perform animal experiments;
- article 9 describes the required scientific background and expertise of people who are allowed to design, coordinate and perform animal experiments;
- article 12 describes the background and expertise of people who are allowed to handle and treat experimental animals (biotechnicians) and to take care of experimental animals (zootechnicians);
- article 14 describes the required scientific background and expertise of people who are allowed to control those that perform animal experiments or handle experimental animals within a licensed institution and monitor animal welfare. The German word *Tierschutzbeauftragter* describes best the function of article 14 officers: people who try to protect animals against unwanted use;
- In article 18 the functioning of the local ethical committees are described.

There are numerous national schools and university courses in which students with a Master's degree in Medicine, Veterinary Medicine, Biology or Dentistry, or researchers with the same background, can obtain an article 9 degree (FELASA, http://www.felasa. org/recommendations.htm). Article 12 officers (biotechnicians) need a lesser education to follow a course.

Case Studies

Three case studies are provided in this chapter. Detailed information can be found in the papers that are listed in the references.

Case 1: Animal Model of Selective Coronary Atherosclerosis[6]

Aim

Development of an animal model that mimics coronary artery stenosis.

Methods

An animal model of selective coronary atherosclerosis was developed by combining a guide-wire induced endothelial injury with administration of a cholesterol-enriched diet. Twelve pigs were subjects of a guide-wire induced endothelial injury of the left anterior descending coronary artery (LAD). Six animals (control group A) were fed a standard pig food diet; the remaining six animals (cholesterol group B) were fed a 6% cholesterol-enriched diet. Three animals from the control group were terminated immediately after the endothelial injury was performed (acute control group A_0). The other three animals from the control group (chronic control group A_4) and all animals from the cholesterol group were terminated four weeks after the endothelium was injured. Histological examination of the LAD and LCX was performed in all groups with light microscopy, scanning and transmission electron microscopy.

Results

The endothelial surface and the media of the LCX were intact in all animals from both control and cholesterol groups. Long eccentric areas of endothelial injury due to the introduction of the guide-wire were found in the LAD in the acute control group. Fibrous atherosclerotic plaques in LAD were found in the chronic control group, as well as in the cholesterol group, but were more pronounced in the latter group. Lipid accumulation (e.g. foam cells) was not found in the plaques of both groups.

We concluded that administration of a 6% cholesterol diet for a period of six weeks is not sufficient to develop coronary atherosclerosis in pigs. Selective coronary atherosclerosis can be induced within four weeks with the same diet when the blood vessel has been injured mechanically with a guide-wire.

Case 2: Animal Model for Tracheal Research[7]

Tracheal research covers two main areas of interest: tracheal reconstruction and tracheal fixation. Tracheal reconstructions are aimed at rearranging or replacing parts of the tracheal tissue using implantation and transplantation techniques. The indications for tracheal reconstruction are numerous: obstructing tracheal tumors, trauma, post-intubation tissue reactions, etc. Although in the past years much progress has been made, none of the new techniques have resulted in clinical application at a large scale. Tissue engineering is believed to be the technique to provide a solution for reconstruction of tracheal defects. Although developing functional tracheal tissue from different cultured cell types is still a challenge.

Tracheal fixation research is relatively new in the field and concentrates on solving fixation-related problems for laryngectomized patients. In prosthetic voice rehabilitation, tracheo-esophageal silicon rubber speech valves and tracheostoma valves are used — often accompanied by many complications. The animal models used for tracheal research vary widely, and in most publications proper scientific arguments for animal selection are never mentioned. The reviewed literature showed that the choice of animal models is a multi-factor process in which non-scientific arguments tend to play a key role.[7]

Problems of fixation to the surrounding tissue are a major drawback in the use of the shunt valve, HME (heat and moisture exchange) filters, and especially the tracheostoma valve. To solve these problems, different *tissue connectors* were developed (titanium and silicone rubber rings, surrounded by a mesh made of titanium or polypropylene fibers). The main objective was to test the feasibility of the implantation of these prototypes in a new animal model. Here we discuss the results, problems and complications of the selected Saanen goat model.

In this prospective laboratory study 19 healthy adult female Saanen goats (*Capra hircus*) were used and observed post-surgically

Table 3.   Results of Isolated Coronary Artery Injury Combined with Cholesterol Enriched Diet on Histology

	Control Group A ($n = 6$)			Cholesterol Group B ($n = 6$)	
	Acute Control Group A_0 ($n = 3$)	Chronic Control Group A_4 ($n = 3$)			
Experiment type	acute	chronic		chronic	
Diet	normal	normal		6% cholesterol	
Coronary artery	LAD	LAD	LCX	LAD	LCX
Guide-wire endothelial injury	yes	yes	no	yes	no
Smooth muscle cell proliferation	no	yes	no	yes	no
Formation of connective tissue	no	yes	no	yes	no
Lipid accumulation	no	no	no	no	no

for 12 weeks. Selection criteria such as comparable anatomy and easy handling were used for animal model development. Also a literature search using the Pubmed, Medline and Cochrane library databases was performed. The anatomy of the Saanen goat was investigated in a separate post-mortem study. Surgery consisted of a laryngo-tracheal separation and implantation of a tracheo-esophageal tissue connector and tracheostoma tissue connector with fibrin tissue glue.

Post-operative care consisted of frequent stoma care, monitoring appetite, weight, vital signs and administration of antibiotics, analgesics and mucolytic agents. All animals survived the surgical procedure. However, postoperative care was extensive, labor-intensive and accompanied by several complications. Eleven animals died before the end of the experiment. Due to a percutaneous connection in relative mobile tissue, the tracheostoma tissue connector caused signs of local infection in all cases. There was no evidence of infection around the tracheo-esophageal tissue connector in 18 cases. It was concluded that the use of goats in this tracheostoma model has shown major complications and should therefore only be used for short-term experiments with intensive care.

Case 3: Development of an Animal Model of Acute Ischemic Heart Failure[8,9]

Aim

Development of an reproducible animal model that mimics acute ischemic heart failure in humans.

Methods

Ligation of one or more branches of the coronary artery system often leads to ventricular fibrillation and unwanted death of animals. Heart failure was induced under open chest conditions, by combining partial ligation of the left circumflex coronary artery (LCX) with cardiac pacing techniques in sheep ($n = 3$). Cardiac pacing resulted in an increased oxygen demand, especially during post-occlusive reactive hyperaemia. Partial ligation prevented the coronary arteries from dilating, resulting in episodes of severe ischemia, in turn resulting in elevated S-T segments.

Results

Pacemaker-induced tachycardia combined with mild coronary artery occlusion resulted in a decrease in aortic pressure from 97 to 70 mm Hg. Left ventricular end diastolic pressure increased from 14 to 27 mm HG; stroke volume decreased from 58 to 43 ml; myocardial segment length shortening decreased from 19% to 16% in the left anterior descending coronary artery supply area, and from 18% to 14% in the LCX (circumflex) area.

Conclusions

These three case studies demonstrate that it is difficult to mimic clinical conditions *in-vitro*. The animal experiments, however, contributed to a better understanding of the processes studied. In all three of the experiments, alternatives could not be found that would made these experiments unnecessary.

References

1. Zutphen LFM van, Baumans V, Beynen AC (eds.). (2001) *Principles of Laboratory Animal Science: A Contribution to the Humane Use and Care of Animals and the Quality of Experimental Results.* Elsevier Science Publishers, Amsterdam, pp. 202–3.
2. Gross D. (1994) *Animal Models in Cardiovascular Research.* Kluwer Academic Publishers, pp. 3–4.
3. http://www.ahc.umn.edu/rar/refvalues.html
4. http://www.thepetcenter.com/exa/nv.html
5. www.ahc.umn.edu/rar/cagespace.html
6. Mihaylov D, Van Luyn MJ, Rakhorst G. (2000) Development of an animal model of selective coronary atherosclerosis. *Coron Artery Dis* **11**:145–9.
7. Ten Hallers EJO, Rakhorst G, Marres HA, *et al.* (2004) Animal models for tracheal research. *Biomaterials* **25**:1533–43.
8. Li Z, Gu YJ, Cheng QY, *et al.* (2005) Hemodynamic support with the pulsatile catheter pump in a sheep model of acute heart failure. *Artif Organs* (submitted).
9. Mihaylov D, Reintke H, Blanksma P, *et al.* (2000) Development of acute ischemic heart failure in sheep. *Int J Artif Organs* **23**:325–30.
10. Mihaylov D, Rakhorst G, Van der Plaats A, *et al.* (2000) *In vivo* and *in vitro* experience with the PUCA-II, a single-valved pulsatile catheter-pump. *Int J Artif Organs* **23**:697–702.
11. Zo doende (2004), Registry of the Netherlands Food Safety Authorities/animal experiments and experimental animals.
12. Ottesen JL, Weber A, Gürtler H, Mikkelsen LF. (2004) New housing conditions: improving the welfare of experimental animals. *ATLA 2004*, 32 (supplement 1) 397–404.
13. Baumans V, www.vet.uu.nl/viavet/viavet_english/S

Chapter 4

Technology Assessment

*J.M. Hummel**

Health care technologies have the potential to increase life expectancy and improve the quality of life of the general public. The general public has high expectations of these technologies and places more and more demands on the effectiveness of these technologies.[1] In recent decades, however, the increased use of health care technology has increased health care expenditures. Technologies that failed have sometimes shown disastrous effects on health outcomes. In response to these impacts on society, an increasing amount of research has focused on the systematic evaluation of the effects of health care technology.

Health Care Technology Assessment

Health care technology assessment (HCTA) is the assessment of the medical, economic, social, legal, ethical, and organizational effects of the application of health care technology. Its outcomes intend to influence clinical and policy decision-making. These decisions often concern the choice to apply a new technology in health

*Science Technology Health and Policy Studies School of Management and Governance University of Twente, Postbus 217, 7500 AE Enschede, The Netherlands.

care, or to withhold a technology from clinical practice. Generally, the medical technology under assessment has completed its development process, and is being used in clinical practice.[2] In this clinical practice, information is gathered to evaluate the effects of the application of this technology.

Methods of Health Care Technology Assessment

Health care technology assessments can roughly be divided into two categories; studies related to the efficacy of a new technology and studies related to the effectiveness. The efficacy-related studies are generally conducted in the early stages of the application of a new technology in clinical practice: when the technology has been used to treat a limited number of patients. These studies focus on clinical outcomes, which include the **efficacy and safety** of a health care technology — whether a given technology can, at least under ideal circumstances, improve some people's health.[3] The effectiveness-related studies are often applied in later stages of clinical application. These studies focus on the **effectiveness** of a technology — whether including it in the repertoire of health care improves people's health under ordinary circumstances, in ordinary settings.[3] This effectiveness is compared with alternatives; whether it generally improves health more than alternative technologies or other health care interventions.

Efficacy Analysis

The most dominant method to measure the efficacy of health care technology is the **randomized controlled trial**. New technologies are tested on people after laboratory and animal studies show promising results. Study participants are randomly allocated among treatment and control group in these experimental studies.[3] Those in the experimental group get the medications or treatments being tested, while those in the control group get a standard treatment or no treatment. Random allocation is intended to ensure that all comparison groups are reasonably similar not only with regard to known characteristics, but also to unknown characteristics that might influence the outcome. All clinical trials are controlled based on a protocol. A protocol describes which people may participate in the trial, as well as the procedures, test schedules, medications and dosages, and the length of the study. Participants are monitored regularly to determine the safety and efficacy of their treatment.

The type of effects generally evaluated in a clinical trial will be illustrated here by a well-known example concerning the St Jude mechanical heart valve. Endocarditis, an infection at the inner side of the heart, is an infrequent but life-threatening complication of cardiac valve replacement. In order to prevent this complication, the cuff of the St Jude heart valve is coated with silver. This element is an agent that reduces bacterial colonization. The seemingly innocent product modification seemed to evoke, however, serious complications. A data safety monitoring board suspended a large-scale clinical trial.[4] The silver-coated valves evidenced a higher risk of infection, thrombus formation, and leakage between the cuff and heart tissue than those without the coating did. As a result, the worldwide clinical inventory of this type of heart valve was recalled in 2000. As shown in this example, clinical trials generally study the medical effects of a new or modified technology. The outcomes may have a strong influence on clinical practice.

Cost-Effectiveness Analysis (CEA)

The most common study in this category is the cost-effectiveness analysis. **Cost-effectiveness analysis** is a structured comparative evaluation of two or more health care interventions.[5] It compares the ratio between the cost and value of one technology with an alternative health care intervention. It calculates, for example, the cost per lives saved. This ratio of the costs and effects of the technology is then compared with ratios from other interventions. Data about the economic and medical effects of the technology can often be found in administrative databases or can be derived by means of questionnaires.

An example of a cost-effectiveness analysis is a health care technology assessment of liver transplantation. An assessment was conducted to decide if liver transplantations should be included in common clinical practice.[6] Medical data about the life-years gained were derived from clinical databases. Data about the quality of these life-years were asked for by means of questionnaires. The costs, including labor costs of the medical profession, stay at the hospital. The costs of the facilities, such as the operating theater and instruments, products and medicine used were found in the administration system. One year after the transplant, most survivors experienced a virtually normal quality of life. The cost-effectiveness ratio was estimated at 21,000–60,000 euro per life-year gained. This ratio was compared with the cost-effectiveness ratio of the regular care of liver patients that does not include a liver transplant. This comparison turned out to be in favor of liver transplantation. Nevertheless, since the effectiveness of liver transplantation in the long term was not yet known, and its cost-effectiveness ratio was lower than the ratio of heart transplants, the decision to include liver transplantation in common practice was postponed. This example shows that assessments focused on the effectiveness of a technology analyze a broader range of effects than the efficacy studies. These effects include medical, economic and social effects. Moreover, this example shows that this cost-effectiveness study of liver transplantation, just like cost-effectiveness studies on heart transplantation and in-vitro fertilization[7] was not used to actually change clinical practice.

The examples in this chapter illustrate the Collingridge dilemma. When the technology is in an early stage of clinical application, the information is often restricted to medical effects. When the technology is in an advanced stage of application, the available information is more comprehensive, yet the assessment's influence on changing the established clinical practice meets more resistance.[8] At this time, the efficacy of the technology has already been shown, and the technology is often already well accepted in the medical profession. Consequently, changing the nature of the technology or influencing its application is difficult at that time.

Constructive Technology Assessment

Constructive technology assessment (CTA) aims to estimate the technology's effectiveness *before* its clinical introduction. Instead of trying to change an already established clinical application of health care technology, methods of constructive technology assessment attempt to influence the development process of health care technologies.[9] Its outcomes can support the people that are involved in the development and clinical application of a technology to improve the technology's effectiveness at the time it is still under development.[10,11]

Methods of Constructive Technology Assessment

CTA assesses and improves the effectiveness of a technology through discussions between technology producers and users and external groups. Technology producers are the medical industry and universities that develop the technology. Users may be medical specialists and nurses, the managers that facilitate the use of the technology, technicians that maintain the technology, and patients that are treated by the technology. The external groups include governments, unions and pressure groups. Methods of CTA facilitate discussions between these groups. They include consensus development conferences, social experiments, and dialogue workshops.[9] In general, these CTA methods have been applied at a national level to create awareness in society about the possible consequences of using new technology.

This chapter emphasizes a practical method of CTA that directly influences the development activities of the technology under assessment. This method involves systematic discussions between the diverse people involved in technological development and clinical application, quantitatively supported by a technique for decision analysis. This method is illustrated by a case study about a medical blood pump, the PUlsatile CAtheter pump (PUCA pump). The assessment was used to determine whether this technology was either acceptable or unacceptable for tests involving patients, or required design modifications.

A Constructive Technology Assessment
of the PUCA Pump

The PUCA pump

The PUCA pump is a blood pump that provides temporary support (hours to a week) to a failing heart (see Fig. 1). It consists of an extra-corporeally placed membrane pump connected to a valved polyurethane catheter. By means of a guiding catheter, the tip of the catheter is introduced via peripheral arteries or open thorax into the left ventricle. The pump aspirates at least 3L/min of blood from the left ventricle and ejects it into the aorta.[12] The PUCA-pump project was at the time of the study focusing on in-house product testing in order to conclude the technology development activities.

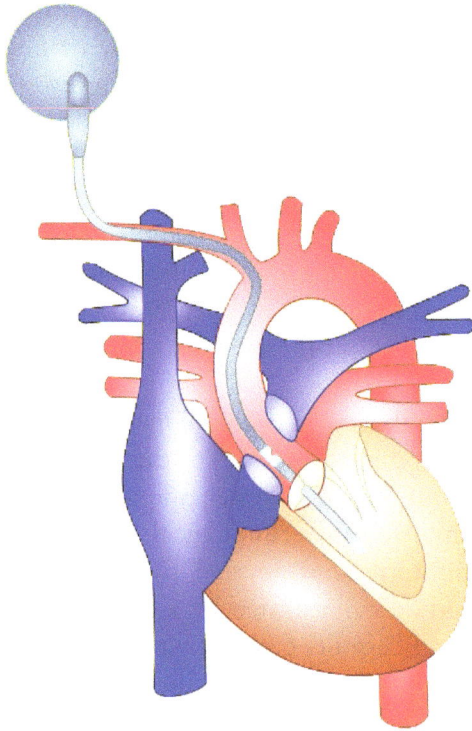

Fig. 1.   PUCA pump.

Methodology

The main experts engaged in the activities related to research and development, manufacturing and future application of the PUCA pump conducted the technology assessment. These medical specialists and engineers were supported by an independent facilitator. In this assessment, the effectiveness of the PUCA pump was being compared to the effectiveness of two alternative blood pumps used in clinical practice: the intra-aortic balloon pump (IABP) and the hemopump, which is a ventricular impeller pump.

Prior to the assessment, every evaluator had received factual information about the characteristics of the new technology and its two competitors. The first stage of the assessment was a brainstorming session about the technology requirements that might be relevant, such as safety and functional requirements. These requirements were divided into main and sub-requirements. Discussions focused on the importance of these requirements and on how effective the three blood pump were in fulfilling these requirements. Explicit attention was paid to the discussion of differences in judgments between the participants. Weighting factors for the requirements and priorities for the trans-arterial blood pumps were computed following the mathematical procedures of the analytic hierarchy process. (See for information about this mathematical technique for decision analysis: Saaty, 1989[13]; and its application in health care: Hummel *et al.*, 2000[10,11]). In the final stage of this assessment, discussions took place about these results and the possibilities to improve the effectiveness of the PUCA pump.

Results

Figure 2 shows the assessment structure of the PUCA pump, consisting of the main requirements imposed upon the blood pumps, the sub-requirements, and the alternative blood pumps: the IABP and the hemopump. The 15 sub-requirements relate to the main requirements: pump performance, safety, ease of use and applicability. In addition, the costs involved in applying the blood pumps were analyzed.

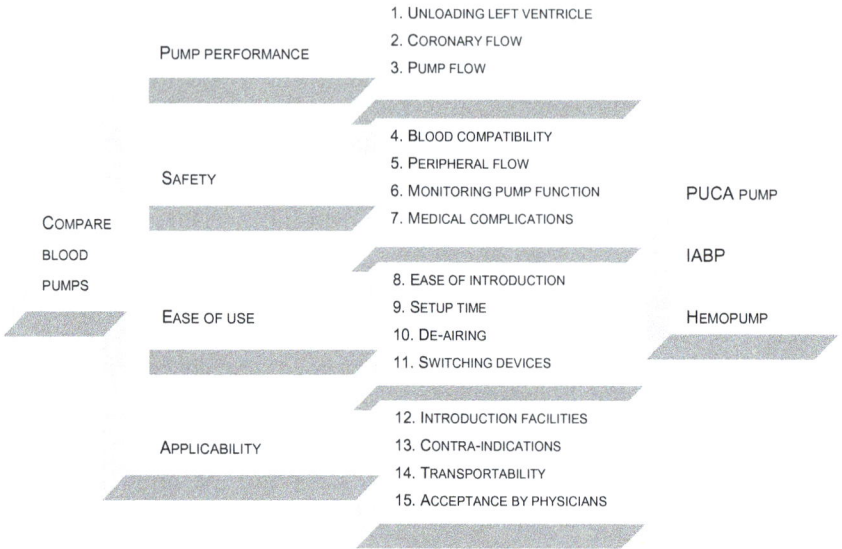

Fig. 2.   The assessment structure of the PUCA pump.

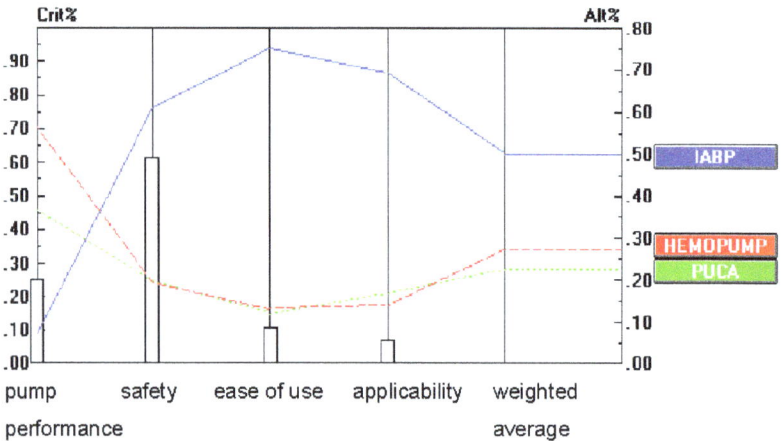

Fig. 3.   Main results of the PUCA pump assessment.

Figure 3 represents the main results of the PUCA pump assessment. It shows the effectiveness of the alternative blood pumps in fulfilling the main requirements. The importance of the main requirements is represented in the height of the bars. Safety is, for example, considered to be the most relevant requirement. The heights of the lines represent the relative effectiveness of the blood pumps in fulfilling these requirements. It shows, for example, that the pump performance in order of decreasing performance is the hemopump, PUCA pump and the IABP. The overall weighted averages show that the IABP is considered to be the most effective blood pump. Even though it has a relatively low pump performance, it is a relative safe pump due to its less intensive contact with blood.

These results indicated that the development process of the PUCA pump needed adjustments. One option was to improve the overall effectiveness to such an extent that the PUCA pump becomes a viable alternative to the IABP. Central in this case are improvements with respect to safety, including modifications of the design of the pump to allow peripheral flow, and the introduction of a training program. Another option is to restrict the clinical application of the PUCA pump to those medical indications that particularly attune to the properties of the PUCA pump. Most importantly, the pump performance of both the PUCA pump and the hemopump is considerably higher than the pump performance of the IABP. Therefore, the PUCA pump could more adequately support a patient group for which pump performance is crucial. Currently, an improved version of the PUCA is being tested in patients. The first patient tests showed that the PUCA pump can be safely applied to support the heart with a blood flow of 2.5 L/min.[14]

Discussion

Randomized controlled trials are important for technology planning — to plan which technology to include in the general practices of health care. The results of randomized controlled trials are relatively reliable. Due to the randomized study design and the strict protocols, the certainty that the treatment actually caused the effects is high. A disadvantage is that the strict trial protocols limit the generalizability of the trial. Moreover, it is expensive and administratively difficult to run randomized trials. They often are narrowly focused on medical effects. The possibility to include more effects would increase the expense and practical difficulties of such large scale experiments. But when ethical and practical reasons allow a randomized controlled trial, it is nonetheless well established as the method of choice.

Cost-effectiveness analyses provide essential additional information about the effects of medical technology and are therefore essential for technology monitoring, to monitor the effectiveness of health care technology used in clinical practice over a longer period of time. The range of effects analyzed is generally broader than that in randomized controlled trials. Therefore, more relevant effects that need consideration are studied. Since the technology is applied under realistic circumstances, the outcomes are relatively generalizable to common practice. A drawback is that changing clinical practice often meets strong resistance. While efficacy studies, such as the study about the heart valve, have a direct influence on clinical decision-making, the impact of cost-effectiveness studies, such as in the case of liver transplantation, on clinical practice is limited. Moreover, when the design or application of the technology is modified, the HTA outcomes may no longer be applicable.

CTA is important to improve technology development. It supports an analysis of the effectiveness of a new technology before clinical application, or of a modified version of a technology already used in clinical practice. During a CTA, the technology developers and the future users of the health care technology discuss the effectiveness and possibilities to improve the effectiveness of the technology. Discussions between these physicians and technological engineers are pivotal. The physicians often possess in-depth knowledge about the requirements to impose on the technology, as well as the effectiveness of existing technological solutions, while the engineers are more knowledgeable about new technological solutions. Moreover, involving the patients, clinicians, technological developers, and manufacturers in the assessment can evoke innovative ideas to improve the effectiveness of the technology. In addition, the discussions help to solve disagreements about the effectiveness of the technology under assessment. This, in combination with the early timing of an assessment, before the technology's clinical application, make it more likely that the suggested modifications are actually implemented to prevent later clinical failure.

CTA analyses a broader range of effects than the efficacy and even effectiveness studies do. In the CTA of the PUCA pump, clinicians, technological developers, and manufacturers formulated the requirements they deemed relevant. Regarding the PUCA pump, these requirements were related to the product's or technology's safety, function, user friendliness, clinical applicability, and costs. As is the case for many health care technologies, safety was regarded to be the most important consideration, to be followed by the main function of the device. The remaining factors are important to take into account as well, such as the ease of use. This is one of the factors that is likely to determine that a technology will actually be used in clinical practice. The predicted effectiveness of the PUCA pump regarding all these medical, technical, social and economic effects guided the technological developers to modify the design and the medical indications for using the blood pump.

Such an evaluation does not, however, imply that all future complications can be predicted. The experiences with the silver-coated heart valve might be a cautious tale about the unknown uncertainties involved with technological advances. The value of CTA lies in reducing the uncertainties that can be recognized by the diverse relevant experts. In the case of the heart valve, this would consider the field of ion beam-assisted coating technology, the toxicity of the coating, or the bio-adhesion to the coating. Even before clinical use, it creates a more comprehensive awareness of the effectiveness of a technical design and design modifications in order to prevent later clinical failure. A drawback of CTA is that the subjective predictions of experts are not as reliable as the objective evidence derived from clinical practice, as used in the efficacy and effectiveness studies. Yet CTA can be a valuable addition to these studies by improving technological development.

References

1. Kumar A. (1999) Management of health care technology literature (1979–1997): a multidimensional introspection. *IEEE Trans Eng Manag* 46(3):247–64.
2. Banta HD, Luce BR. (1993) *Health Care Technology Assessment and its Assessment, an International Perspective*. Oxford University Press, Oxford.

3. U.S. Congress, Office of Technology Assessment. (1994) *Identifying Health Technologies that Work: Searching for Evidence.* U.S. Government Printing Office, Washington DC.
4. Schaff H, Steckelberg JM, Grunkemeier GL, Holubkov R. (1999) Artificial valve endocarditis reduction trial (AVERT): protocol of a multicenter randomized trial. *The Journal of Heart Valve Disease* 8(2):131–9.
5. Drummond MF, Stoddard GL, Torrance GW. (1987) *Methods for the Economic Evaluation of Health Care Programmes.* Oxford Medical Publications, Oxford.
6. Bonsel GJ, Habbema JD, Bot ML, *et al.* (1989) Technology assessment of liver transplantation; a study of the liver transplantation program in Groningen 1977–1987. *Nederlands Tijdschrift der Geneeskunde* 133(28):1406–14.
7. Rossum W van. (1991) Decision-making and medical technology assessment: three Dutch cases. *Knowledge and Policy* 4:1–2.
8. Collingridge D. (1980) *The Social Control of Technology.* Francis Pinter, London.
9. Schot JW, Rip A. The past and future of constructive technology assessment. *Technological Forecasting and Social Change* 54:251–68.
10. Hummel JM, Rossum W van, Verkerke GJ, Rakhorst G. (2000) Medical technology assessment: the use of the analytic hierarchy process as a tool for multidisciplinary evaluation of medical devices. *Int J Artif Org* 23(11):782–7.
11. Hummel JM, Rossum W van, Verkerke GJ, Rakhorst G. (2000) Assessing medical technologies in development; a new paradigm of medical technology assessment. *Int J Tech Assessment Health Care* 16(4):1214–9.
12. Verkerke GJ, Muinck ED de, Rakhorst G, Blanksma PK. (1993) The PUCA pump: a left ventricular assist device. *Artif Org* 17(5):365–8.
13. Saaty TL. (1989) Group decision-making and the AHP. In: Golden BL, Wasil EA, Harker PT. (eds.), *The Analytic Hierarchy Process; Applications and Studies,* Springer-Verlag, Berlin.
14. Grandjean J, Kuipers MJ, Warkotsch G, Mariani M. (2005) Use of the PUCA pump during beating heart surgery. *NVT.*

Chapter 5

Haemocompatibility of Medical Devices

*W. van Oeveren**

The use of blood-contacting biomaterials is increasing yearly by 12%. Biomaterials are used for implants (stents, heart valves, vascular grafts), for temporary support or monitoring in the body (infusion systems, catheters, drug delivery, heart pumps), or for extracorporeal circulation (dialysis, apheresis, heart-lung machine). In most situations a proper anticoagulation is essential to prevent immediate thrombosis. However, much more knowledge about blood-material interactions must be obtained to reduce other side effects, such as micro-thrombosis and an inflammatory reaction. Those who are involved in the construction of medical devices should be aware of the response of platelets, coagulation, and complement immediately after contact with a biomaterial. Furthermore, they should realize that haemocompatibility of the biomaterial is of major concern for uneventful use of a device. This should be verified with proper testing. Progress is being made with different types of coating, which might be used to cover even the most thrombogenic surface.

*Department of BioMedical Engineering, University Medical Center Groningen, A. Deusinglaan 1, 9713 AV Groningen, The Netherlands.

Introduction

The number of serious adverse events induced by blood-contacting devices is increasing due to an increased number of applications and new products. Consensus exists on the important role of poor haemo-compatibility in direct and sustained adverse reactions. Therefore, understanding and prevention of uncontrolled blood-material inter-actions is pivotal for safe use of blood-contacting devices. Some of the most studied effects of biomaterials in contact with blood will be discussed in this chapter. Application of biomaterials in direct blood contact results in activation of the blood coagulation system and in an inflammatory reaction. These responses of blood are due to the natural response of the host defense mechanism against for-eign surfaces. This may result in pathological processes, such as microthrombi generation, thrombosis, bleeding complications, haemodynamic instability, fever, edema, and organ damage. These adverse events become manifest during prolonged and intensive foreign material contact with vascular implants and extracorporeal blood circulation.[1,2]

Surface Interactions of Blood

After contact of blood with a material, various proteins will be deposited within split seconds (see Fig. 1). The main proteins adhered to a surface are albumin, fibrinogen and immunoglobulin, based on their high concentrations in blood (see Table 1). After the initial adhesion a continuous exchange with free proteins takes place, which reaches equilibrium after approximately two hours. This results in binding of higher-molecular weight proteins. The rel-atively medium-molecular weight protein albumin will be exchanged in part for larger proteins. Next to non-specific protein deposition, some components of the contact system react specifically with negatively charged surfaces. As soon as the blood comes in con-tact with a negatively charged foreign surface, Factor XIIa frag-ments are formed. These fragments then initiate the entire contact system. β-Factor XIIa converts prekallikrein into its active form,

Blood -Material interaction

Protein deposition

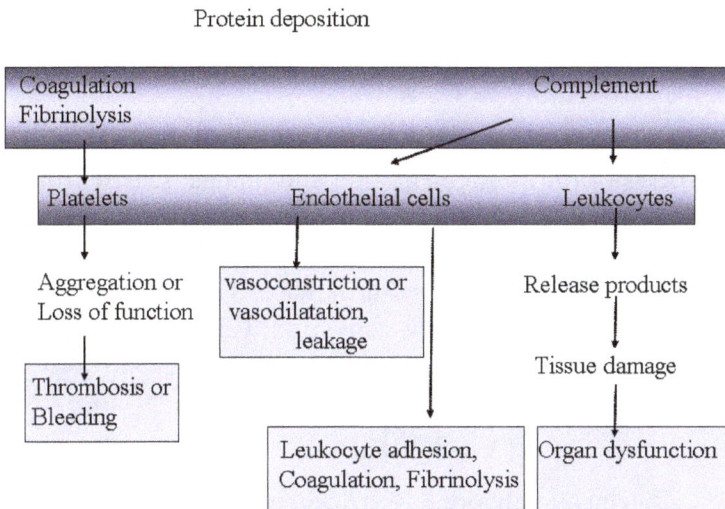

Fig. 1. Proteins of the clotting cascade and complement bind immediately during blood contact of a biomaterial. The number of activating proteins and the conformational change after binding determine to what extent platelets, endothelial cells and leukocytes will be involved in the reaction. Finally thrombosis, bleeding, altered blood pressure, and inflammation may occur after activation of the various cascades.

Table 1.   Blood Composition

Plasma 60%	Cells 40%
Albumin (40 g/L)	Erythrocytes (8 μm) $4300 \cdot 10^9$/L
Globulins $\alpha+\beta+\gamma$ (30 g/L)	Platelets (3 μm) $200 \cdot 10^9$/L
Fibrinogen (3 g/L)	Leucocytes (10 μm) $5 \cdot 10^9$/L

kallikrein, which generates the vasodilator bradykinin.[3] The deposition and conformation of some plasma proteins on the artificial surface, such as Factor XII, fibrinogen and vitronectin are a significant criterion for further thrombogenicity.[4] After deposition to some surfaces, fibrinogen leads to a strong adhesion of platelets through platelet glycoprotein receptors (GpIIbIIIa), followed by platelet aggregation and release of procoagulant contents from platelets. Additionally, contact activation induces activation of the coagulation cascade (see Fig. 2).

Fibrin clots and thrombi are cleared by fibrinolysis, the enzymatic process of fibrin fragmentation and platelet release from binding to fibrinogen. The fibrinolytic enzyme, plasmin, can be formed through either the release of endothelial tissue plasminogen activator (t-PA) or by kallikrein-activated urokinase. The inflammatory reaction is initiated by complement activation. C3b, which is present in

Coagulation

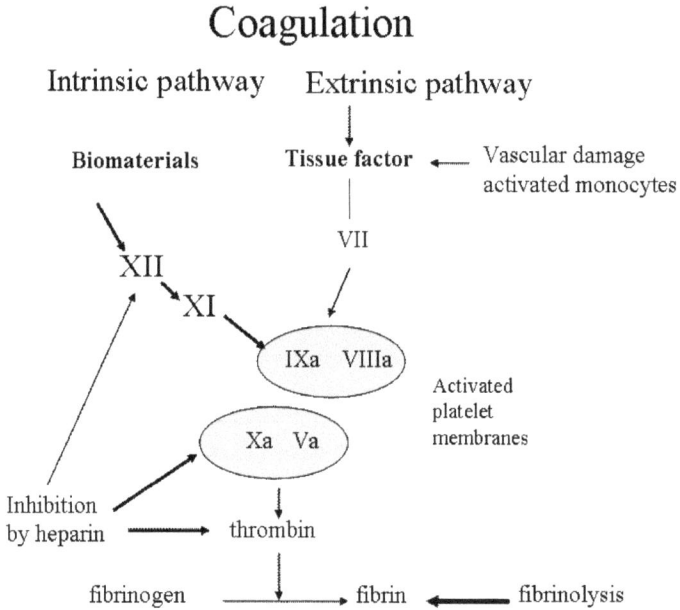

Fig. 2.   The main products involved in coagulation, including the intrinsic and extrinsic pathway. Although the intrinsic pathway has physiologically almost no meaning, it plays an important role in activation by biomaterials. The intrinsic pathway is initiated by the contact system (XII and kallikrein) or by Factor XI. Deposition of leukocytes results, among other things, in tissue factor activation, whereas activated platelet membranes contribute to coagulation by complex formation of factors IX, VIII, X and V.

small amounts in blood, after adhesion to a negatively charged surface, forms a C3 convertase (C3 cleaving enzyme) when not immediately degraded by complement inhibitors. Since foreign surfaces lack complement inhibiting capacity, the complement convertases will amplify the complement reaction by cleavage of new C3 molecules, resulting in C3b generation and its deposition onto the surface.

Simultaneously, the smaller C3a fragment is released in plasma, and this fragment is often used as a marker of complement activation. Thus, an exponential activation of the complement system takes place after recruitment of the other complement factors (see Fig. 3). Similarly to C3 convertase, C5 convertase will also be formed, with cleavage capacity for C5 into C5a and C5b conversion. Complement

Complement pathways

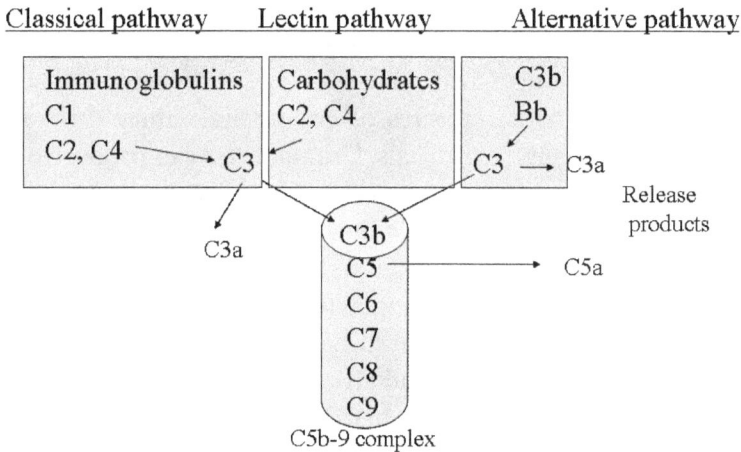

Fig. 3. The alternative pathway of the complement system reacts independently of other immune factors on any foreign surface by deposition of factor C3b and subsequent recruitment of other factors, such as Bb. The C3 convertase cleaves new C3 molecules to form C3b and C3a, which enhances deposition of C3b and causes signaling of leukocytes by release of C3a and C5a. Finally, the terminal complement complex, composed of all factors C5b-C9, is formed. This complex may cause cell lysis.

has lytic effects on target cells by its end stage components, C5b-9 (terminal complement complex), and therefore may become harmful for the patient in contact with an activating device. Moreover, most of the deleterious effects of complement activation are related to the recruitment and activation of leukocytes, such as granulocytes and monocytes. Granulocytes show an upregulation of the adhesion molecules CD 11 and CD 18 with increased adhesion to the surface, release of elastase and superoxide generation, i.e. further propagation of the inflammatory response.[5,6]

Leukocytes

Leukocytes release a number of inflammatory products including chemotactic factors, growth factors, and complement components. A second mechanism involves the production of lysosomal degradation enzymes. Activated leukocytes elaborate several potent proteases capable of degrading collagen and other structural extracellular matrix and extracellular components, for example, basement membranes. Heparanases can remove heparan sulphate proteoglycans from the cell surface and diminish their inhibition on cell proliferation.[7] Lastly, leukocytes may also act at sites of endothelial injury through the production of oxygen free radicals. Granulocytes can produce oxygen free radicals capable of injuring remaining viable endothelium, leading to an ongoing stimulation of inflammatory injury.[7,8]

Inflammatory processes related to biomaterials have been studied extensively in patients undergoing extracorporeal circulation (heart-lung machine or dialysis). During surgery and the early post-operative stage, the extent of the inflammatory response is associated with clinical symptoms such as fever, bleeding and, in severe cases, organ failure.[2,9] This is more pronounced after use of the heart-lung machine, due to its large surface area and corresponding massive activation of the complement system.

Platelets

Platelets are essential to stop bleeding because they bind to the subendothelium of a damaged blood vessel, aggregate to form a plug and stimulate local coagulation. Platelet adhesion to subendothelium requires the interaction of the platelet receptor GpIb, plasma von Willebrand factor and fibronectin. Platelet adhesion to biomaterials occurs by binding to fibrinogen and GpIIbIIIa. Platelet aggregation requires fibronectin, von Willebrand factor or vibronectin, and most often platelet receptor GpIIbIIIa. The adhered platelets release adenosine diphosphate and activate the arachidonic acid synthesis pathway to produce thromboxane A2.[10] Thromboxane A2 is a potent chemoattractant and smooth muscle cell mitogen, and leads to further platelet recruitment.[11] Once activated, platelets release constituents of their granules. Upon activation, and during apoptosis, platelets and other cells bud off small parts of their plasma membrane, called microparticles (MP).[12]

> Platelets are most important for thrombosis and clotting in flowing blood.

A specific platelet activation, e.g. on biomaterials, can have opposite effects: thrombi may be formed by circulating platelet aggregates and bleeding may occur due to loss of functional platelets. Therefore, a lot of effort is made to prevent platelet activation by biomaterials.

Biomaterials in Clinical Practice

Small implants in the blood vascular system: stents and vascular grafts. After balloon dilatation of narrowed small-diameter arteries, stents are frequently applied to maintain the lumen open. The basis material of stents is a metal, such as stainless steel, tantalum, or nitinol, based on the mechanical properties of these metals to support the vascular wall with minimal occlusion of side branch capillaries. The occurrence of in-stent subacute thrombosis has been reduced, but still remains as a worrying complication because of its strong impact on short-term mortality.[13] Due to the refinement of adjunctive antiplatelet treatment[14] and the establishment of the most appropriate ways for stent utilization,[15] reduced thrombosis was observed around the turn of the millennium.

However, an increase of thrombotic incidents has been observed since, due to increased stent utilization, and also related to new types of bioactive coatings, aiming to reduce the late reappearance of a coronary stenosis at the site of intervention (restenosis) due to intimal hyperplasia. The triggers for the formation of intimal hyperplasia that have been further defined are growth factors, injury, circulating blood components, and haemodynamics.[16,7,17] Implantation of a medical device into the arterial circulation leads to endothelial denudation, which is immediately followed by deposition of platelets and leukocytes. Besides damage to the endothelium, high arterial pressure and flow cause damage to the medial layer of the blood vessel. In particular, biomaterial implants with poor haemocompatibility and poor rheology will cause platelet activation and the subsequent release of platelet-derived growth factor.[18]

Extracorporeal Circulation

In 2004, almost 700,000 heart operations worldwide were performed with the assistance of extracorporeal circulation (ECC). The possibilities of operating on these patients successfully can be explained by continuous improvement in operative techniques, as well as perioperative supervision and mechanical circulatory support systems. The optimization of the surfaces of ECC devices is of increased importance, both during the operation (heart-lung machine) and after operation with systems providing sustained heart support. Next to the technical perfection of all these systems, it is also particularly important to consider the surfaces presented to the circulating blood. Insufficient haemocompatibility of materials used for ECC devices still remains a problem. The contact between blood and the various artificial surfaces of the corporeal system leads post-operatively to a post-pump syndrome, which can escalate into a systemic inflammatory response syndrome (SIRS),[19] acute lung failure (ARDS, adult respiratory distress syndrome),[20] sepsis, or even multi-organ failure (MOF).[21] The causes of these syndromes are multi-factorial: mechanical and chemotactic activation and membrane-damage of the blood cells, dysfunction of cellular immune regulation, and activation of the haemostatic system.

The materials used for extracorporeal application include a wide spectrum of polymers, in particular polyethylene, polypropylene, polyvinylchloride, polyester, polystyrene, polyurethane and silicone. Although these products possess the required physical properties, they display more or less the same disadvantage: an incompatibility with blood and tissues. Through contact with the blood this incompatibility can provoke a pathophysiological response from the organism, similar to that of traumatic shock. As is well known, in adult patients undergoing a bypass grafting procedure, the total blood volume comes into contact with about $3\,m^2$ of these non-physiological surfaces for one to several hours. This extensive contact causes a massive activation of the humoral and cellular defense systems. Such side effects of biomaterials are counteracted in part by coating surfaces to obtain improved biocompatibility or by pharmacological inhibition of the enzymes responsible for consecutive activation of the cascade reactions.

Biomaterial Surface Characteristics in Relation to Haemocompatibility

Minimal generation of thrombosis is a very important requirement for biomaterials used for temporary support of organs or as permanent implants in the human body. Adhesion and activation of platelets to biomaterials surfaces is an important step in thrombosis and is governed, in part, by surface energy and wettability of the biomaterial surface.[22] Prior to adhesion of platelets, plasma proteins like fibrinogen and fibronectin adsorb,[23] and the composition of the adsorbed plasma proteins relates to the wettability of the biomaterial surface.[24] Adhesion can be controlled by adjusting the surface properties — especially surface energy — of the material involved.

> Implants with poor haemocompatibility remain a pathogenic factor a long time.

Long-term implantation of totally artificial hearts is one of the most compelling proofs of the bio-engineering utility of surface energy modification to minimize biological adhesion. These pumps, and the related intra-aortic balloons and left ventricular assist devices, do not accumulate blood clots or thrombotic masses during their contact with blood.

Wettability

Wettability indicates the behavior of water on a surface: a high wettability is water-friendly (hydrophilic) and will result in the spreading of a drop of water on the surface. A low wettability is hydrophobic and results in round water droplets on the surface. Albumin, fibrinogen and immunoglobulin G are the most prevalent proteins in blood plasma[25] and their adsorption is higher on hydrophilic materials. Generally, more platelets adhere to hydrophilic than to hydrophobic material, while flow promotes platelet adhesion, evidently through increased convective mass transport.[26] A moderate flow and shear stress (0.8 N/m^2) generated the most pronounced difference in platelet adhesion between hydrophilic and hydrophobic surfaces. However, when the flow was further increased to simulate the conditions of coronary arteries at 3.2 N/m^2, platelet numbers at the hydrophilic end were significantly reduced as compared with the hydrophobic end. These results strongly suggest detachment of platelets from hydrophilic surfaces.

Such effects can be explained by the small contact area of platelets with hydrophilic surfaces.[27] Furthermore, the platelets attached to hydrophilic surfaces remain spherical and, extend deeper into the blood flow, thereby experiencing higher shear forces. In contrast, platelets on hydrophobic materials can withstand high shear forces due to strong contact and complete spreading of platelets. When examined with scanning electron microscopy, the platelets on the hydrophobic end of a gradient surface were indeed more extended like a pancake than on a hydrophilic end.[28] Obviously, platelets behave opposite to water in contacting hydrophilic or hydrophobic surfaces. Thus, in high-flow (arterial) areas hydrophilic surfaces will accumulate fewer platelets, as will hydrophobic surfaces in low-flow areas.

Roughness

The influence of biomaterial roughness on thrombogenicity is not clear, since various studies show apparently conflicting results. Angiographic catheters with different surface roughness were most thrombogenic when the surface was smoothest, whereas surface chemistry (polyethylene versus polyamide) contributed to a lesser extent to thrombogenicity.[29] Increased roughness caused a decrease in platelet adhesion on hydrophilic surfaces and an increase on hydrophobic surfaces. These results were obtained when flow conditions were applied. During static test conditions no differences between smooth and rough surfaces were found.[30,31]

One explanation for different observations is the higher extent of thrombogenicity at smooth surfaces, whereas the degree of thrombus adhesion is higher at rough surfaces.[32] In a more detailed study it was observed that roughness due to titanium crystals appeared to initiate more activation of the clotting cascade, but less platelet adhesion.[33] These different effects of two important factors of thrombus formation in conjunction with the variability induced by various flow and shear stress conditions and wettability may explain the conflicting results regarding the thrombogenicity of biomaterials.

Haemocompatibility of Polymers and Metals

Due to their mechanical and radio-opaque properties metals are frequently used for manufacturing implant devices and as part of devices used for invasive procedures for diagnostic and therapeutic purposes. Often, these implants are in direct contact with blood, e.g. as stents, heart valves and catheter tips. The blood compatibility data of metals are relatively scarce, which is possibly due to the historically accepted application of metals as medical devices, or to the indispensable physical characteristics of metals. Most frequently used metals even appear to have prothrombotic properties, which, if alternatives were available, would lead to refusal of their use in blood-contacting devices or implants. No thorough comparisons between metals can be made, since most studies report only limited blood compatibility tests. Apparently, the possible induction of an inflammatory reaction, initiated by complement activation or granulocyte activation, is not frequently tested, although it is an important contributor to intimal hyperplasia.[34]

It can be concluded that the more noble metals appear less haemocompatible than oxidized titanium and aluminum metals (ceramics) and silicon carbon products. Most bare metals have a poor haemocompatibility in direct comparison to polymers. Some of the most frequently used polymers and metals are discussed here.

Polymers

The polymers commonly used for manufacturing medical devices, such as PVC, polyethylene, polyurethane and polycarbonate have good haemocompatibility if no monomers or additives are leaching from the end product. The use of PVC is under debate for its high concentration of phthalate plasticizers (up to 40%), which accumulate in the environment and have negative effects on the reproductive system.

Metals

Stainless steel — stainless steel (316L) is the most commonly used metal for endovascular devices. Its mechanical properties significantly contribute to its applicability, but the blood compatibility results also appear better than those of some other metals. For instance, stainless steel stents are more blood compatible than tantalum stents.[35] However, stainless steel can also be further optimized, since several studies have showed that polymer coating of stainless steel stents reduced deposition of platelets and thrombus mass by more than 60%.[36] The clotting system is activated significantly by stainless steel.

Metals without coating have a poor haemocompatibility.

Tantalum — After stainless steel, tantalum was introduced as the preferred metal for the construction of stents. Implantation of tantalum stents is greatly facilitated by tantalum's high radiopacity. Initial studies showed similar blood compatibility for tantalum and stainless steel,[37] although later studies indicated that stainless steel possesses better blood compatibility.[35] Clinical studies indicated that a high incidence of thrombotic complications could occur after tantalum stent implantation if anticoagulation and antiplatelet therapy was insufficient.[38] Also, post-stent antithrombotic therapy was required, including both anticoagulants and platelet inhibitors, or Ticlopidine plus Aspirin.[39] Polymer coating of tantalum stents with polyurethane or parylene reduced the deposition of platelets by 5% to 50% relative to platelet deposition on uncoated stents.[40]

Titanium and Nitinol — In the human body, titanium exists only for a short period of time in its unmodified form, and relevant blood compatibility data are therefore obtained with titanium nitride or titanium oxide. Titanium oxide appears to reduce fibrinogen deposition due to its semi-conductive nature. This effect is explained by the similar electronic structures of fibrinogen and titanium.[41] In a comparative study with low-temperature isotropic pyrolytic carbon (L TI carbon), it not only reduced deposition of fibrin, but also resulted in a 50% reduction in microscopically counted platelets with titanium oxide.[42] Transvenous inferior vena-cava filters made of stainless steel, titanium or titanium-nickel all showed approximately 25% early thrombosis in clinical use, measured via ultrasound scanning.[43] This incidence of early thrombosis was unexpectedly high, and difficult to reduce with the current devices, since antithrombotic medication is often contra-indicated in patients requiring a vena-cava filter.

Titanium nitride has been tested for its blood compatibility with regard to leukocyte adhesion, and appears to retain no leukocytes.[44] *In vivo* experiments with titanium nitride heart-valves in sheep showed some deposition of fibrin and platelets.[45]

Nickel-titanium alloy (Nitinol) has attracted special attention due to its shape memory function. It must be noted that Nitinol has an outer surface of titanium (oxide), whereas nickel is not exposed to blood. Therefore, blood compatibility characteristics are expected to be rather similar to those of titanium oxide.

Biological Surface Treatment to Improve Haemocompatibility

Materials with good haemocompatibility have a preference for binding with albumin. Albumin has been described to inhibit the release reaction of platelets and to inhibit platelet aggregation.[46] Fibrin deposition and platelet receptor-binding was also reduced on tubing of an extracorporeal system after pre-coating with albumin. However, the initial albumin coating will be replaced by other proteins during prolonged blood contact as a result of the Vroman effect.[47]

A further improvement of surfaces requires a more irreversible surface treatment. Depending on the treatment, the surface may be modified to induce less thrombogenic or inflammatory reactions. Heparin, cell membrane phospolipids and block copolymer coatings are often used on a number of blood contacting devices. Most of the pioneering work was done with extracorporeal systems, by which adverse effects of blood-material contact are most obvious.

Heparin Coating

After the first heparin-coated extracorporeal circuits became available in the last half of the 1980s, their haemocompatibility was shown in *in vitro* systems, animal models and patient studies.[48] It can be concluded that heparin-coated circuits can cause a reduction of activation of the contact phase, complement system activation, inflammation and pulmonary complications.[49,50] The reduced thrombogenicity of the heparin-coated surfaces was thought to be attributable to the inhibition of thrombin by catalyzing the binding to antithrombin III. However, more recent data show that the advantage of heparin coating lies much more in the reduced, or selective, adhesion of plasma proteins. This leads to a faster formation of a blood-friendly secondary layer and prevents a further denaturation, and hence activation, of the adhered proteins and blood cells.

Phosphorylcholine Coating

Phosphorylcholine-containing lipids dominate in the outer membrane of the cell membrane bilayer, and these appear to possess strong antithrombotic properties.[51] One such lipid allows the coupling of synthetic methacryloylphosphorylcholine/lauryl-methacrylate copolymers to metal and synthetic surfaces. The term biomembrane mimicry arose for phosphorylcholine-coated foreign surfaces.[52] *In vitro* experiments and animal tests have shown that phosphorylcholine-coated artificial polymers possess outstanding thrombogenic resistance and display only minimal adhesion of plasma proteins and platelets.[53] This coating technique has been offered for, among others, contact lenses, stents and extracorporeal circulation devices.

In vitro experiments showed decreasing complement activation with increasing surface phosphorylcholine mole fractions,[54] suggesting that phosphorylcholine is responsible for the reduction. The working mechanism is probably related to lesser activation of the complement protein C5[55] and the inhibition of monocyte and macrophage adhesion.[56]

SMA Coating

Surface modifying additives (SMAs), are mixed with the initial synthetic materials in the production phase, and this technique is therefore not a coating in the usual sense. The copolymer distributes itself in the synthetic materials during the polymerization process and, due to its charge characteristics, moves to the surface of the basis material as it cools. Thus, a new surface of primarily SMA forms. The microscopic structure of the surface of alternating hydrophilic and hydrophobic regions carries a zero net charge, thereby reducing platelet and leukocyte deposition. Tsai *et al.*[57] proved that SMA surfaces decreased coagulation activation and significantly reduced contact phase and complement activation. Gu *et al.*[58] found better platelet protection in clinical CPB by using SMA-treated devices. However, larger clinical studies on routine cardiopulmonary bypass patients showed only minor clinical benefits of SMA-treated devices.

PMEA Coating

Poly-2-methoxyethylacrylate (PMEA) is a hydrophilic polymer coating that minimizes the adsorption and denaturation of proteins and blood cells. In various animal and clinical studies, this coating has been proven to reduce blood activation during extracorporeal circulation. Plasma bradykinin levels and the percentages of activated monocytes in PMEA-coated circuits were significantly lower than those in uncoated circuits during CPB. The amount of protein adsorbed on PMEA-coated circuits was 10 times lower than that on uncoated circuits.

A clinical study showed no significant differences between heparin-coated and PMEA-coated groups in the plasma concentrations of inflammatory markers, or markers of clotting. Clinical variables did not differ between the groups. It was concluded that PMEA-coated CPB circuits are as biocompatible as heparin-coated CPB circuits and prevent post-operative organ dysfunction in patients undergoing elective coronary artery bypass grafting with CPB.[59] The cost-effectiveness ratio seems favorable for PMEA-coated circuits.[60]

> The best choice of biomaterial (wettability, roughness), depends on its application; in fast, slow, or non-circulating blood, different requirements apply.

Testing of Medical Devices

In December 2002 the revised ISO 10993-Part 4 standard (*Biological evaluation of medical devices — Selection of tests for interactions with blood*) was published.[61] The standard is applicable to external communicating devices, either with an indirect blood path (e.g. blood collection devices, storage systems) or in direct contact with circulating blood (e.g. catheters, extracorporeal circulation systems), and implant devices (stents, heart valves, grafts). Testing should be performed for five categories, based on primary processes: thrombosis, coagulation, platelets, haematology and complement. In this system all relevant aspects of blood activation are taken into consideration, and testing should simulate clinical conditions as much as possible.

One important aspect of testing of medical devices is the condition of blood exposure to the device. Therefore, anticoagulation and flow conditions must be as similar as possible to the clinical application to achieve relevant test results. Thus, most devices must be tested with heparinised blood under circulating conditions. For some devices, such as stents and catheters this implies high flow through or around the device to obtain relevant shear stress conditions. The major differences observed between cell interaction under static and flow conditions has made clear that whole-blood flow models are required for testing haemocompatibility inasmuch as the test device will be used clinically in the blood circulation. Flow models for testing may consist of animal models or *in vitro* test systems. Animal models have the advantage of the more physiologic condition and the important antithrombotic effects of endothelial cells. A disadvantage is the higher costs and often insensitivity due to overwhelming short-term effects of tissue damage. Moreover, it has been shown that the composition of blood differs considerably between various species, which leads to over- or under-estimation of human blood reactions to biomaterials.[62,55] The use of human blood is therefore more relevant to the interpretation of results and offers a more detailed array of test methods, since most available methods are based on human-blood components. The use of human blood requires a proper *in vitro* circulation model.

The rheological properties of blood influence the adhesion of platelets and the capture and adhesion of leukocytes, as well as their margination in the bloodstream.[63] Increasing erythrocyte aggregation correlates with increasing leukocyte adhesion and with more slow-flowing leukocytes near the wall. Thus flowing erythrocytes promote leukocyte adhesion, either by causing margination of leukocytes or by initiating and stabilizing the attachment that follows.

Clinical examples of situations of a marked change in rheology are intense blood loss and subsequent replacement with clear solutions[64] and the use of a heart-lung machine for cardiopulmonary bypass (CPB). During CPB a number of non-physiological events take place including haemodilution, hypothermia, and non-pulsatile flow. As a consequence of these events rheology changes and blood flow may be stimulated to shunt from a less-favored organ to preserve a more vital organ.[65] During CPB, the intestines and kidneys are suffering from this altered rheology. Increasing concentrations of damage markers have been found during and after CPB.[66] During rewarming additional damage may occur.[67] A haematocrit value below 25% is a primary risk factor in developing severe renal dysfunction.[68]

> Testing of a blood-contacting product should be done under conditions that mimic the final clinical application.

When blood is in contact with biomaterial surfaces, fluid mechanics, and especially the shear stress, have a strong influence on the damage of red cells and platelets. Red cell damage may occur at high shear stress.[69,2] Platelets are more easily damaged by shear stress.[2] Platelet damage is not only influenced by the maximum shear, but also by the duration of the shear force. Only for very short exposure times are platelets able to withstand higher shear stress than red cells.[70]

From a fluid-mechanical point of view, differences in flow situations may therefore lead to different problems with blood. Artificial heart valves may cause problems for red cells due to the short duration of very high shear,[2] whereas stents in the coronary arteries induce intimal growth at locations of relatively low shear,[71] which may be caused by platelet activation in high shear. Neointima formation in stents has been shown to be related to wall shear stress as well.[71] In tubing used during dialysis, the high shear rate at the needle may lead to problems for red cells,[72] but it should not be disregarded that the wall shear stress of the tubing is the most critical issue for platelet activation.

Heart valves, extracorporeal systems and vascular grafts or stents induce relatively high shear forces, which may result in platelet activation. Shear stress is a natural activator of platelets. The shear-induced pathway appears to be one of the major pathways of platelet induced haemostasis and thrombosis.[73]

A classical *in vitro* test model is the Chandler loop,[74] which consists of a closed tube partly filled with air, which circulates the device constantly with an air-liquid interface at low shear rates only. This method also may induce artifacts due to the major forces applied on blood elements and to protein denaturation at the air-liquid interface.[75] Thus, instead of the Chandler loop a small roller pump closed-loop system was used in the past. This model appeared effective for short-term circulation.[35] However, blood damage induced by the pump limited the exposure of the test object to circulating blood. Since improvement of the model by minimizing blood damage may increase sensitivity and permits prolonged blood exposure,[76] a simple mechanical device without air and without a pump to reduce blood damage and activation by the device was constructed. Moreover, the new device provided pulsatile flow at a frequency similar to the arterial circulation. This Haemobile induced less intrinsic blood damage than the Chandler or roller pump and was most suitable for testing of thrombosis induced by tubing, arterial stents and mechanical heart valves.[77]

Conclusion

In spite of all the technical improvements on the haemocompatibility of biomaterials, a noticeable activation of plasma proteins and corpuscular blood components still exists. The long-range aim remains the creation of an optimally haemocompatible surface (endothelium-like), which blood would no longer recognize as unphysiological, and hence would not induce humoral and cellular defenses, or the rejection mechanisms against it.

On-line monitoring of organ damage (point of care testing) is essential in order to apply optimized conditions. The currently used markers of organ dysfunction are too non-specific or too much dependent on an advanced stage of deterioration of the organ. Therefore, newer, sensitive organ damage markers for early organ damage will probably be introduced in routine practice. Bare metal parts exposed to blood should be avoided, either by coating, oxidation or replacement by haemocompatible polymers. Further, the blood composition in terms of haematocrit and plasma expanders should be optimized, to ensure proper oxygen delivery to all organs.

An important new item is compliance with magnetic resonance imaging (MRI) techniques, which will be a common method of screening for malignancies, inflammatory sites and infarctions. Stainless steel and nickel could particularly raise problems in MRI scans.

Finally, thorough haemocompatibility testing should have a prominent place in the certification of blood-contacting medical devices, since a poor haemocompatibility has long-lasting negative effects on the whole body, through blood transport of activation products, and on functional recovery at the site of implant.

References

1. Kirklin JK, Westaby S, Blackstone EH, *et al.* (1983) Complement and the damaging effects of cardiopulmonary bypass. *J Thorac Cardiovasc Surg* **86**: 845–57.
2. Yoganathan AP. (1995) Cardiac valve prostheses. In: Bronzino JD, ed. *The Biomedical Engineering Handbook*, CRC Press, Boca Raton, Florida, pp. 1847–70.
3. Mammen EF. (1990) Contact activation: the interaction of clotting, fibrinolytic, kinin and complement systems. *Biomed Prog* **2**:31–4.
4. Vroman L. (1998) The life of an artificial device in contact with blood: initial events and their effect on its final state. *Bull NY Aead Med* **64**:352–7.

5. Moen O, Hogasen K, Fosse E, *et al.* (1997) Attenuation of changes in leukocyte surface markers and complement activation with heparin-coated cardiopulmonary bypass. *Ann Thorac Surg* **63**:105–11.

6. Wan S, LeClerc JL, Vincent JL. (1997) Inflammatory response to cardiopulmonary bypass: mechanisms involved and possible therapeutic strategies. *Chest* **112**:676–92.

7. Ip JH, Fuster V, Badimon L, *et al.* (1990) Syndromes of accelerated atherosclerosis: role of vascular injury and smooth muscle cell proliferation. *JACC* **15**:1667–87.

8. Davies MG, Hagen PO. (1994) Pathobiology of intimal hyperplasia. *Br J Surg* **81**:1254–69.

9. Moat NE, Shore DF, Evans TW. (1993) Organ dysfunction and cardiopulmonary bypass: the role of complement and complement regulatory proteins. *Eur J Cardiothorac Surg* **7**:563–73.

10. Brass LF. (1991) The biochemistry of platelet activation. In: Hoffman R, Benz EI, Shattil SJ, Furie B, Cohen HJ. (eds.), *Hematology. Basic Principles and Practice*, New York, Edinburgh, London, Melbourne, Tokyo, Churchill Livingstone, pp. 1176–97.

11. Bassiouny HS, Song RH, Kocharyan H, *et al.* (1998) Low flow enhances platelet activation after acute experimental arterial injury. *J Vasc Surg* **27**:910–18.

12. Tans G, Rosing J, Thomassen MC, *et al.* (1991) Comparison of anticoagulant and procoagulant activities of stimulated platelets and platelet derived microparticles. *Blood* **77**:2641–8.

13. Kobayashi Y, De Gregorio J, Kobayashi N, *et al.* (1999) Comparison of immediate and follow-up results of the short and long NIR with Palmaz-Schatz stent. *Am J Cardiol* **84**:499–504.

14. Colombo A, Hall P, Nakamura S, *et al.* (1995) Intracoronary stenting without anticoagulation accomplished with intravascular ultrasound guidance. *Circulation* **91**:1676–88.

15. Balcon R, Beyar R, Chierchia S, *et al.* (1997) Recommendations on stent manufacture, implantation, and utilisation. Study Group of the Working Group on Coronary Circulation. *Eur Heart J* **181**:536–47.

16. Davies MG, Hagen PO. (1995) Pathophysiology of vein graft failure. *Eur J Vasc Endovase Surg* **9**:7–18.

17. Newby AC, Zaltsman AB. (2000) Molecular mechanisms in intimal hyperplasia. *J Path* **190**:300–09.

18. Ross R, Raines EW, Bowen-Pope DF. (1986) The biology of platelet-derived growth factor. *Cell* **46**:155–69.

19. Taylor KM. (1996) SIRS — the systemic inflammatory response syndrome after cardiac operations. *Ann Thorac Surg* **61**:1607–8.

20. Müller E. (1991) Adult respiratory distress syndrome (ARDS): activation of complement, coagulation and fibrinolytic systems. *Biomedical Progress* **4**:3–6.

21. Colman RW. (1995) Hemostatic complications of cardiopulmonary bypass. *Am J Hematol* **48**:267–72.
22. Baier RE. (1984) Adhesion in the biologic environment. *Biomater Med Dev Artif Organs* **12**:133–59.
23. Harmand MF, Briquet F. (1999) *In vitro* comparative evaluation under static conditions of the hemocompatibility of four types of tubing for cardiopulmonary bypass. *Biomaterials* **20**:1561–71.
24. Tsai CC, Deppisch RM, Forrestal LJ, *et al.* (1994) Surface modifying additives for improved device-blood compatibility. *ASAIO J* **40**:M619–24.
25. Warkentin P, Wälivaara B, Lundström I, Tengvall P. (1994) Differential surface binding of albumin, immunoglobulin G and fibrinogen. *Biomaterials* **15**:786–95.
26. Spijker HT, Graaff R, Boonstra PW, *et al.* (2003) Review: on the influence of flow conditions and wettability on blood-material interactions. *Biomaterials* **24**:4717–27.
27. Spijker HT, Bos R, Van Oeveren W, *et al.* (2002) Adhesion of platelets under flow to wettability gradient polyethylene surfaces made in a shielded plasma. *J Adhesion Sci Technol* **16**:1703–13.
28. Spijker HT, Bos R, Busscher HJ, *et al.* (2002) Platelet adhesion and activation on a shielded plasma gradient prepared on polyethylene. *Biomaterials* **23**:757–66.
29. Bailly AL, Lautier A, Laurent A, *et al.* (1999) Thrombosis of angiographic catheters in humans: experimental study. *Int J Artif Organs* **22**:690–700.
30. Zingg W, Neumann AW, Strong AB, *et al.* (1982) Effect of surface roughness on platelet adhesion under static and under flow conditions. *Can J Surg* **25**:16–19.
31. Zingg W, Neumann AW, Strong AB, *et al.* (1981) Platelet adhesion to smooth and rough hydrophobic and hydrophilic surfaces under conditions of static exposure and laminar flow. *Biomaterials* **2**:156–8.
32. Hecker IF, Edwards RO. (1981) Effects of roughness on the thrombogenicity of plastic. *J Biomed Mater Res* **15**:1–7.
33. Maitz MF, Pham MT, Wieser E, Tsyganov I. (2003) Blood compatibility of titanium oxides with various crystal structure and element doping. *J Biomater Appl* **17**:303–19.
34. Miller DD, Karim MA, Edwards WD, Schwartz RS. (1996) Relationship of vascular thrombosis and inflammatory leukocyte infiltration to neointimal growth following porcine coronary artery stent placement. *Atherosclerosis* **124**:145–55.
35. Monnink SH, Van Boven AJ, Peels HO, *et al.* (1999) Silicon-carbide coated coronary stents have low platelet and leukocyte adhesion during platelet activation. *J Investig Med* **47**:304–10.

36. Seeger M, Ingegno MD, Bigatan E, *et al.* (1995) Hydrophilic surface modification of metallic endoluminal stents. *J Vasc Surg* 22:327–36.
37. Scott NA, Robinson KA, Nunes GL, *et al.* (1995) Comparison of the thrombogenicity of stainless steel and tantalum coronary stents. *Am Heart J* 129:866–72.
38. Hamm CW, Beytien C, Sievert H, *et al.* (1995) Multicenter evaluation of the Strecker tantalum stent for acute coronary occlusion after angioplasty. *Am Heart J* 129:423–9.
39. Park SW, Park Sl, Hong MK, *et al.* (1997) Coronary stenting (Cordis) without anticoagulation. *Am J Cardiol* 79:901–04.
40. Fontaine AB, Koelling K, Passos SD, *et al.* (1996) Polymeric surface modifications of tantalum stents. *J Endovasc Surg* 3:276–83.
41. Nan H, Ping Y, Xuan C, *et al.* (1998) Blood compatibility of amorphous titanium oxide films synthesized by ion beam enhanced deposition. *Biomaterials* 19:771–6.
42. Zhang F, Zheng Z, Chen Y, *et al.* (1998) *In vivo* investigation of blood compatibility of titanium oxide films. *J Biomed Mater Res* 42:128–33.
43. Aswad MA, Sandager GP, Pais SO, *et al.* (1996) Early duplex scan evaluation of four vena cava interruption devices. *J Vasc Surg* 24:809–18.
44. Dion I, Roques X, More N, *et al.* (1993) *Ex vivo* leukocyte adhesion and protein adsorption on TiN. *Biomaterials* 14:712–19.
45. Mitamura Y, Hosooka K, Matsumoto T, *et al.* (1989) Development of a ceramic heart valve. *J Biomater Appl* 4:31–55.
46. Kottke-Marchant K, Anderson JM, Umemura Y, Marchant RE. (1989) Effect of albumin coating on the *in vitro* blood compatibility of Dacron arterial prostheses. *Biomaterials* 10:147–55.
47. Vroman L, Adams AL, Fischer GC, Munoz PC. (1980) Interaction of high molecular weight kininogen, factor XII, and fibrinogen in plasma at interfaces. *Blood* 55:156–9.
48. Wendel HP, Ziemer G. (1999) Coating-techniques to improve the hemocompatibility of artificial devices used for extracorporeal circulation. *Eur J Cardiothorac Surg* 16:342–50.
49. Boonstra PW, Gu YJ, Akkerman C, *et al.* (1994) Heparin coating of an extracorporeal circuit partly improves hemostasis after cardiopulmonary bypass. *J Thorac Cardiovasc Surg* 107:289–92.
50. Gu YJ, Van Oeveren W, Van der Kamp KWHL, *et al.* (1991) Heparin coating of extracorporeal circuits reduces thrombin formation in patients undergoing cardiopulmonary bypass. *Perfusion* 6:221–5.
51. Zwaal RFA, Comfurius P, Van Deenen LLM. (1977) Membrane asymmetry and blood coagulation. *Nature* 268:358–60.
52. Chapman D, Lee DC. (1987) Dynamics and structure of biomembranes. *Biochem Soc Trans* 15:475–545.

53. Von Segesser LK, Tonz M, Leskosek Band Turina M. (1994) Evaluation of phospholipidic surface coatings *ex vivo*. *Int J Artif Organs* **17**:294–8.
54. Ishihara K, Nakabayashi N. (1995) Hemocompatible cellulose dialysis membranes modified with phospholipid polymers. *Artif Organs* **19**:1215–21.
55. Salerno CT, Droel J, Bianco RW. (1998) Current state of *in vivo* preclinical heart valve evaluation. *J Heart Valve Dis* **7**:158–62.
56. DeFife KM, Yun JK, Azeez A, *et al.* (1995) Adhesion and cytokine production by monocytes on poly(2-methacryloyloxymethyl phosporylcholine-co-alkyl methacrylate)-co polymers. *J Biomed Mat Res* **29**:431–9.
57. Tsai WB, Grunkemeier JM, Horbett TA. (1999) Human plasma fibrinogen adsorption and platelet adhesion to polystyrene. *J Biomed Mater Res* **44**:130–9.
58. Gu YJ, Boonstra PW, Rijnsburger AA, *et al.* (1998) Cardiopulmonary bypass circuit treated with surface-modifying additives: clinical evaluation of blood compatibility. *Ann Thorac Surg* **65**:1342–7.
59. Ninomiya M, Miyaji K, Takamoto S. (2003) Influence of PMEA-coated bypass circuits on perioperative inflammatory response. *Ann Thorac Surg* **75**:913–17.
60. Saito N, Motoyama S, Sawamoto J. (2000) Effects of new polymer-coated extracorporeal circuits on biocompatibility during cardiopulmonary bypass. *Artif Organs* **24**:547–54.
61. *ISO 10993 Biological Evaluation of Medical Devices — Part 4: Selection of Tests for Interactions with Blood*, Dec 2002.
62. Bodnar E. (1996) The Medtronic parallel valve and the lessons learned. *J Heart Valve Dis* **5**:572–3.
63. Abbitt KB, Nash GB. (2003) Rheological properties of the blood influencing selectin mediated adhesion of flowing leukocytes. *Am J Physiol Heart Circ Physiol* **285**:H229–40.
64. Morariu AM, Maathuis MAJ, Asgeirsdottir SA, *et al.* Acute isovolemic hemodilution triggers proinflammatory and pro-coagulatory endothelial activation in vital organs: role of erythrocyte aggregation. *Microcirculation*, in press.
65. Swan HJC. (1957) Discussion note. *Ann Surg* **146**:560.
66. Morariu AM, Loef BG, Aarts LPHJ, *et al.* (2005) Dexamethasone: benefit and prejudice for patients undergoing on-pump coronary artery bypass grafting. *Chest* **28**:2677–87.
67. Lema G, Meneses G, Urzua Z, *et al.* (1995) Effect of extracorporeal circulation on renal function in coronary surgical patients. *Anesth Analg* **81**:446–51.
68. Ranucci M, Pavesi M, Mazzo E, *et al.* (1994) Risk factors for renal dysfunction after coronary surgery: the role of cardiopulmonary bypass technique. *Perfusion* **9**:319–26.
69. Keller KH. (1981) The dynamics of the interaction of cells with surfaces. In: Salzman EW (ed.), *Interaction of the Blood with Natural and Artificial Surfaces*, Dekker, New York, pp. 119–38.

70. Anderson GH, Heliums JD, Moake J, Alfrey CP Jr. (1978) Platelet lysis and aggregation in shear fields. *Blood Cells* **4**:499–511.
71. Wentzel JJ, Krams R, Schuurbiers JC, *et al.* (2001) Relationship between neointimal thickness and shear stress after Wallstent implantation in human coronary arteries. *Circulation* **103**:1740–5.
72. De Wachter DS, Verdonck PR, Verhoeven RF, Hombrouckx RO. (1996) Red cell injury assessed in a numerical model of a peripheral dialysis needle. *ASAIO-J 1996* **42**:M254–9.
73. Brien JR. (1990) Shear-induced platelet aggregation. *Lancet* **335**:711–3.
74. Chandler AB. (1958) *In vitro* thrombotic coagulation of blood: a method for producing a thrombus. *Lab Invest* **7**:110–16.
75. Ritz-Timme S, Eckelt N, Schmidtke E, Thomsen H. (1998) Genesis and diagnostic value of leukocyte and platelet accumulations around "air bubbles" in blood after venous air embolism. *Int J Legal Med* **111**:22–6.
76. Munch K, Wolf MF, Gruffaz P, *et al.* (2000) Use of simple and complex in vitro models for multiparameter characterization of human blood-material/device interactions. *J Biomater Sci Polymer Ed* **11**:1147–63.
77. Yoshizaki T, Tabuchi N, Van Oeveren W, *et al.* (2005) PMEA polymer-coated PVC tubing maintains anti-thrombogenic properties during *in vitro* whole blood circulation. *Int J Artif Organs* **28**:834–40.

Chapter 6

Tissue and Cell Interactions with Materials

T.G. van Kooten* and R. Kuijer*

Biomaterials serve different purposes in biomedical technology and medicine. In this chapter the reactions of tissues and cells towards biomaterials are described. The focus is on materials that are implanted to support or replace damaged tissue or organs.

The adhesion of cells and tissues to biomaterials is an essential part and determines the overall reaction. Adhesion hardly ever occurs to the materials themselves, but instead to a protein layer covering the materials. The composition of the protein layer, as well as the conformation of the proteins, is determined by the physicochemical properties of the biomaterial surface. Apart from these properties, the tissue/cell response towards degradable and non-degradable materials differs. The foreign-body reaction in particular results in complete removal of the degradable material from the implantation site and subsequent resorption. Non-degradable materials are encapsulated and therefore isolated as a foreign body, although a continuous, mild inflammatory reaction might persist.

*Department of BioMedical Engineering, University Medical Center Groningen, A. Deusinglaan 1, 9713 AV Groningen, The Netherlands.

Materials that are indistinguishable from the bodies' own materials will generally not evoke a foreign-body reaction.

Introduction

Cell adhesion to and growth on biomaterials is an important issue in implantology. Often the final result of this interaction can be witnessed by means of histological evaluation of the tissues that are directly apposing the implant material. A sequence of events occurs in a patient when an implant is positioned and although the sequence and the events can depend on the site of implantation, as well as the application, several common characteristics apply. Furthermore, several steps can be modeled in *in vitro* systems using cell cultures. The aim of this chapter is to highlight the current knowledge on the path from initial cell-material interactions towards integration of the material with surrounding tissues.

(Bio)materials are defined as follows: a material intended to interface with the biological system to evaluate, treat, augment or replace tissue, organ or function of the organism (Chester Conference, 1991). In other words, it is any material used in the body to achieve a therapeutic or diagnostic purpose. It can be used inside the human body as/in: prostheses, matrix material for tissue engineered devices, a capsule for cellular implants, biosensors, and many other applications.

Probing Cell-Material Surface Interactions

Apart from a thorough physico-chemical characterization of the material surface under consideration (see below), it is necessary to analyze the cell response due to interaction with the material surface. In principle, all currently known cell biologic methods can be applied to this area of research. Furthermore, our fundamental understanding of the molecular biology of cells, as described in a number of outstanding textbooks, can be integrated with knowledge about cell behavior at the interface with materials.

> There is no unambiguous reference biomaterial to compare all others with.

Cell attachment and adhesion, two phenomena with distinct features, are usually determined with light microscopy or scanning electron microscopy (SEM) (see Fig. 1). Light microscopic micrographs can be used to quickly assess the cell-surface interaction without understanding the principles of the interaction. Numbers of cells adhered have also been estimated in a comparative way by using DNA assays or so-called cell viability assays in which a compound is converted by enzyme systems to a detectable, colored or fluorescent substance. Examples are MTT, XTT and calcein-AM ester known from the dead-live stains.

The amount of molecules converted within a certain time frame is a measure of the activity of the cultured cells, and cannot always be used to determine adhered cell numbers, as reported in several studies. MTT has also been used to assess proliferation in assays for measuring the effects of drug treatments on cultured cells, and this has been extended to measurements of material-dependent cell proliferation. Due to the general material-dependence of the MTT conversion per cell, this is not legitimate. Other methods to determine proliferation are the 3H-thymidine or BrdU incorporation and Ki67 or PCNA ELISA enzyme-linked immunosorbent assay. In fact, a large number of proteins can be screened in relation to the general control of the cell-cycle as a function of material surface properties. The cycle control includes the process of programmed cell death (apoptosis).

> The binding of cells to materials predominantly occurs through a layer of adsorbed proteins.

The quality of cell adhesion has been determined in many studies in the past 10 years. Although it still is not clear how exactly quality

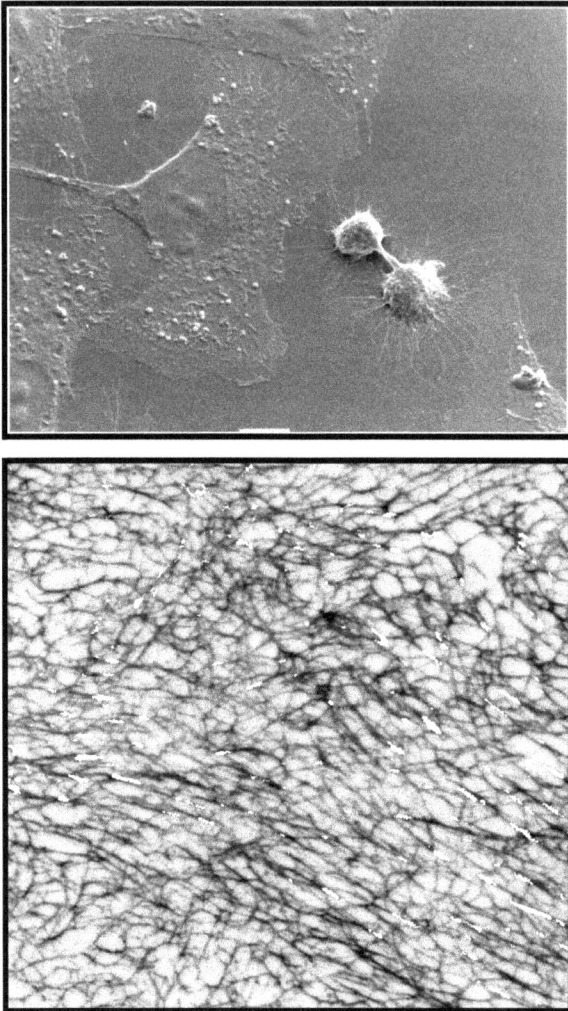

Fig. 1.   Cell-material interactions can be visualized through many microscopic methods, such as scanning electron microscopy (A) and fluorescence microscopy (B). (**A**) Human fibroblasts adhering to polymethylmetacrylate (PMMA). Cells are clearly able to spread. A couple of dividing cells are also present. (**B**) Cells deposit a network of extracellular matrix on the underlying material surface. In this image the fibronectin network is shown deposited by human endothelial cells on tissue culture polystyrene (TCPS). Cells adhere to this matrix through focal adhesions depicted as an overlay of white spots. Besides fibronectin, cells produce other matrix molecules not shown in this image.

should be defined, it is evident that cells need a well-established system of both stress fibers and focal contacts in order to be able to survive and grow. Therefore, in many studies focal adhesion components, as well as actin fibers have been probed with antibody-based detection techniques, such as immunocytochemistry or ELISA. Localization of the proteins concerned is usually done by light microscopy or (confocal laser scanning) fluorescence microscopy (see Fig. 1). Similar determinations have been reported for cell surface receptors involved in cell adhesion. Another approach is the use of assays for determination of the cell binding strength.

The next step to determine the quality of adhesion is to map the signaling pathways involved in transducing the adhesion signals to the nucleus. This is a highly relevant topic because extensive knowledge about the material-dependent regulation of these pathways will allow us to design material surfaces for specific applications.

Apart from adhesion and proliferation, cell function is becoming increasingly important. Function can be probed by methods similar to those described above and relates to functional activities due to cell-substratum interactions and cell-cell interactions while interacting with a surface. Cell-cell interactions, for example, are important for proper communication required in all tissues. Gap-junctional intercellular communications in dermal fibroblasts were supported by hyaluronan polymers consisting of repeating disaccharides of N-acetyl-D-glucoseamine and D-glucuronic acid linked by beta 1–4 glycosidic bonds. Molecular techniques such as the reverse transcriptase-polymerase chain reaction (RT-PCR) and *in situ*-hybridization (ISH) have gained significance in assessing cell function. RT-PCR is a powerful tool for studying the consequences of cell-material interactions at the RNA level as a complementary method for ELISA at the protein level and can be used to obtain (semi-) quantitative data.

One essential problem with studies involving the determination of cell-material interactions remains: there is no unambiguous reference material with which others can be compared. If it is stated that neither excessive migration nor proliferation was found, then it is not clear, nor can it be clear, when migration is excessive. Similarly, it is not always evident what particular data range parameters should have for the most appropriate response. When making comparisons it can be stated that individual cell parameters on one material are higher/lower than on the other, but is much harder to state whether or not this is better. This is exemplified by a study of Groth and co-workers who determined the response of hepatoblastoma cells while interacting with different ultra-filtration membranes. On polyacrylonitrile (PAN) and the hydrophobic polyetherimide (PEI), the cells better expressed focal adhesions and exhibited high growth rates, without adequate albumin synthesis. On the hydrophilic polyacrylonitrile-N-vinylpyrollidone co-polymer (P(AN-NVP)), focal adhesions were less-developed, indicating a weakened cell-substratum adhesion. Furthermore, proliferation decreased. Instead, cell-cell adhesion increased, as did albumin secretion. On the moderately wettable micro-filtration membrane polyvinylidendifluoride (PVDF) the cell-material and cell-cell interactions were poorly developed. Based on these observations, choosing a best polymer cannot be decided without prioritizing the desired parameters of interaction. Solutions to this type of question will appear once our collective knowledge on cell-material interactions and their relevance towards applications further develops. In this respect, the use of high-throughput techniques such as micro-array analysis and proteomics can help us map the genes and the products involved, such as enhanced adhesion or function as a function of polymer surface characteristics. These methods yield a large output of data in terms of numbers of genes and their products being up- or down-regulated. The analysis and validation of these data still is labor-intensive, but nevertheless will speed up our knowledge level on cell-material interactions.

Material Surface Composition

The surface of polymers represents the site at which the interactions take place. Whatever the bulk looks like, a cell will be confronted with a shallow shell of molecules that shape the surface. Physicochemical methods exist to probe the surface for elemental and molecular surface composition, e.g. X-ray photoelectron spectroscopy (XPS) and Fourier transform infrared spectroscopy (FTIR), respectively. This chapter is not meant to deal with these surface characterization techniques, but rather focuses on the results derived from these techniques. The carbon and hydrogen atoms are the main representatives within both the bulk and surface of almost all polymers. Other elements frequently encountered are N, O, F, P and S. Many polymers consisting of C and H atoms do not readily sustain cell adhesion and growth. Therefore, surface modifications have been implemented, which introduce functional groups on the surface that contain any combination of the elements listed above. The effects of these surface modifications can be measured through their interactions with biological systems, including proteins, cells, and microbial organisms. The key issue is to probe what essentially has been altered in favor of a beneficial cell response.

The classic example is the difference between polystyrene (PS) and the tissue-culture variant TCPS. Most adherent cell types do not adhere to PS, but easily adhere to TCPS. Moreover, TCPS generally supports cell spreading and subsequent cell growth very well. In contrast, even if cells attach to PS, cell spreading is very weak, and consequently cell growth is virtually absent. In many studies, TCPS is considered to be the gold standard to which other materials are compared. Although the exact treatment procedure is not publicly known, it is evident that plasma treatment is involved (plasma treatment is also called "radio-frequency glow discharge treatment" or "glow discharge treatment"). This treatment exists in many variations of different kinds of plasma and different conditions that are used during the process. Radio-frequency glow discharge is performed in a vacuum environment with the material in between a cathode and anode. Radical formation at the surface results in the presence of reactive sites that, upon exposure to oxygen (air), allow the formation of covalent bonds with incoming atoms or molecules. Typically, a mixture of hydroxyl ($-CH_2OH$), carboxyl ($-COOH$), carbonyl ($-COOCH_3$), amide ($-CONH_2$) and amine ($-CH_2NH_2$) groups is introduced at the surface.

Depending on the cell type, one particular functional group may be more responsible for the observed, enhanced cell responses than others. Growth of bovine aortic endothelial cells, for example, increased with the surface carbonyl concentration and did not correlate with either hydroxyl or carboxyl groups. Chinese hamster ovary (CHO) cells, on the other hand, showed good adhesion, spreading and growth on a variety of polymers with a high hydroxyl surface density introduced by water vapor plasma treatment. Plasma treatment remains a highly actual topic, as many recent tissue engineering applications require surfaces that sustain cell growth, whereas most of the current degradable materials do not adequately perform this function (see below). Besides plasma treatment, other options exist to create functional polymers carrying chemical functional groups through the macromolecular chains. These options are mainly based on creating reactive groups at the end of the polymer chains that can react with small molecules, which introduce the functional group. Another option is the use of self-assembled monolayers (SAM) with defined terminated groups to create designed functional surfaces. Frequently used contrasting surfaces are carboxylic acid-terminated and methyl-terminated SAMs, providing hydrophilic and hydrophobic surfaces, respectively. Keratinocytes, for example, were shown to adhere and grow well on the acid surface while adhering poorly to the hydrocarbon functionality.

> Biological macromolecules adsorbed to a material surface are influenced by the physical and chemical surface properties.

The atomic and molecular make-up of material surfaces is often reflected in macroscopic surface parameters such as surface charge and wettability. Wettability is a parameter that is usually determined with contact angle measurements of liquid droplets on the material surface. The results are used to indicate the wettability of the surface. This is also referred to as hydrophobicity or hydrophilicity. The contact angles can be converted to interaction energies such as the surface free energy of the material surface and the work of adhesion for approaching cells. Wettability of materials surfaces has been related to cell attachment, cell adhesion and cell spreading.

Exact relationships between cell attachment and surface wettability can be established for a given cell type under a given set of culture conditions. In general terms it can be stated that optimal attachment, spreading and growth occurs at intermediate wettability. Surfaces with a low wettability do not sustain cell adhesion, whereas highly wettable surfaces exhibit cell adhesion to some degree, certainly a higher degree than on the lowly wettable surfaces. The intermediate wettability range is somewhere between 60 and 80 degrees for the water contact angle. It is emphasized that exceptions to this generalized statement exist. Wettability is and will remain a critical material surface parameter for design of new surfaces. Despite clear exceptions to the rule of thumb of an optimum water contact angle window of 60–80 degrees, many researchers use this as a guideline for surface modifications.

The Role of the Extracellular Matrix

Material surfaces can adapt to changes originating from their properties. The biological environment, however, usually influences the surface to a larger extent. Cell attachment to material surfaces is subject to the general, fundamental forces of nature. These include the Van der Waals (London dispersion) and electrostatic forces, as well as hydrogen bonding interactions (also called acid-base interactions, based on protons donating and accepting parts of molecules). Although early attachments can be made with the bare polymer surface, it is highly likely that these attachments will be resolved and replaced by others between the cells and biological compounds. Biological compounds such as proteins adsorb to the surface. This process proceeds much faster and therefore earlier than the cell attachment. Furthermore, almost all cell-containing environments contain these adsorbing molecules. Cell suspensions are often made in a culture medium containing serum components. Materials inserted in the human body come in contact with blood or other tissue fluids with a high content of a huge diversity of proteins. In addition to this, cells will start to produce their own proteins soon after attachment. These include extracellular matrix proteins, such as proteoglycans that are secreted in the surrounding environment (also against the material's surface).

The effect of all these processes is that the naked material surface will soon be masked by a variety of biological macromolecules (see Fig. 1). This has been referred to as a conditioning film in the literature on microbial adhesion. The concept can also be used in the description of cell-material interactions. Conditioning refers to both the modifying and the changing character of the deposited layer.

Despite the masking character of the conditioning film, it has been realized that the underlying material substratum influences the makeup of the biological layer. Already in 1981 materials were classified according to their ability to bind and activate fibronectin. Hydrophobic substrata were shown to activate the cell-binding activity of Fn, whereas hydrophilic surfaces did not. In later studies it was shown that hydrophilic materials bind pre-adsorbed fibronectin that can easily be reorganized into fibrillar structures, whereas on surfaces with water contact angles above 60 degrees cells were not able to do so. In addition, hydrophilic polymer surfaces enhance endogenous fibronectin deposition by cells relative to hydrophobic materials, and only the hydrophilic surfaces support a fibrillar organization of the deposited fibronectin, probably because hydrophobic surfaces do not allow fibronectin exchange from the surface. In many publications the beneficial role of fibronectin in cell growth and function has been described, potentially even wiping out all differences in cell response to surfaces. The presence of some optimum adsorption density seems to apply to fibronectin. Besides fibronectin, other members of the extracellular matrix family can enhance cell adhesion, in particular vitronectin.

A more complex adsorption behavior has been demonstrated with studies involving fibronectin, fibrinogen and vitronectin adsorption out of pure suspensions, full and diluted blood, and (diluted) serum solutions. It has been convincingly shown that polystyrene and TCPS differentially influence fibronectin and vitronectin adsorption from either pure or diluted serum solutions, a phenomenon comparable to the Vroman effect described for a number of proteins adsorbing out of the blood. Differences in adsorption are not so much related to the amount adsorbed, but rather to the quality of the adsorbed molecules, specifically in the exposure of the cell-binding domain. Using antibody detection techniques, several groups have demonstrated that material surfaces influence the exposure of the cell binding domain of fibronectin. Studies on the mechanisms behind this phenomenon are thriving, as a detailed understanding is likely to significantly contribute to a knowledge-based surface design approach.

The modifying effect of adsorbed biological compounds on cell-material interactions relies on specific interactions between the ligands of these compounds and the receptors on the cell membrane. One particular class of receptors can be highlighted for its demonstrated importance in these interactions. The integrins represent a class of currently 20 combinations of alpha and beta chains that combine to cell-surface receptor dimers recognizing a variety of specific sites within extracellular matrix proteins. One of these sites is the amino acid sequence RGD (Arg-Gly-Asp) with flanking residues, which is primarily recognized by the integrin $\alpha5\beta1$. As a result of receptor-ligand binding and integrin cross-linking, signals are forwarded to the cell nucleus resulting in, for example, focal adhesion formation, stress fiber assembly and cell growth. Individual ECM proteins or parts of these proteins can be used as specific absorbing proteins for enhancing cell adhesion. Fibronectin, for example, has often been applied to serve this purpose. Other proteins include laminin, vitronectin and fibrinogen. These adsorbed or covalently coupled proteins are thought to directly influence the makeup of the eventual conditioning film. This concept has opened the way towards including other molecules such as growth and differentiation factors, antibodies and cytokines — in fact, the full spectrum of biologically active, mainly small proteins.

Inflammation is a Fundamental Response of the Body Towards Injury

Probing cell-material interactions in *in vitro* systems is a relatively easy task due to the simplification of the system. The number of biological components is limited and often one or two cell types are involved. Materials, however, ultimately are applied in the body. An entirely different world exists surrounding the implanted materials. Before we can go into more detail on the body response towards the implants, it is necessary to know the fundamental response of the body towards injury in general. This response is often referred to as wound healing, and also as inflammation.

Inflammation is part of the defense mechanisms of our body and as such has been well explained in a number of textbooks on immunology and (patho)fysiology. In this paragraph a synopsis on inflammation is presented.

Inflammation is the response of vascularized tissue to injury. It is a biochemical and cellular process. The essential components are predominantly present in the circulation. The early mediators of inflammation affect the vascular bed in such a way that movement of plasma and blood cells out of the circulation into the tissue surrounding the injury occurs. This exudate serves three functions: defense of the host against invading microorganisms, facilitation of tissue repair, and, ultimately, healing.

Two stages of inflammation can be discerned: acute and chronic inflammation. Injury starts off the acute response. Causes of injury to cells can be multifold. Upon injury, the vascular bed around the site of injury immediately starts to react. An initial constriction of arterioles is followed by vasodilation. The effects are an increased exudation of plasma and blood cells. The classical inflammation signs appear: redness (rubor), swelling (tumor), heat (calor), pain (dolor) and sometimes loss of function (functio laesa). Blood cells are able to migrate across the endothelial cell lining by way of complex interactions between receptors and their ligands. The migration process consists of three consecutive stages: margination, diapedesis and exudation. Once in the tissue, cells and proteins show a concerted action for further orchestration of the inflammation response and interaction with components of the immune response. Two cell types are involved in transmigration towards the tissue. The early cells are neutrophilic granulocytes which ingest (phagocytose) microorganisms, cell debris and dead cells. The late cells are the monocytes/macrophages with a similar function. Phagocytosis is associated with a burst of metabolic activity of the phagocytosing cells, resulting in the production of (highly) reactive oxygen-containing molecules. These molecules, together with lysosomal enzymes, are responsible for the breakdown of phagocytosed debris and microorganisms. They can also be responsible for tissue damage when they are released in the tissue due to death of the phagocytes. Some other cell types can be involved in the inflammation process. Platelets are responsible for stopping the bleeding in a process called coagulation. The cells need the support of three circulation-based protein systems (complement, clotting, kinin) and immunoglobulins. The acute inflammation is restricted in time and usually takes 8–10 days to complete. Inflammation is a response of vascularized tissue to injury and can be associated with the removal of infectious microorganisms. But inflammation also occurs without the presence of bacteria, for example, after a sterile surgical procedure.

> Implantation of a biomaterial is generally accompanied by two types of inflammatory responses, a wound healing process and a foreign body reaction.

When the acute inflammation response is able to resolve the consequences of the injury, i.e. kill microorganisms and remove all debris, the lesion is ready for tissue regeneration or repair, ultimately resulting in wound healing. Although the healing process is governed by the same principles throughout the body, the outcome can be different depending on the site of injury. A myocard infarct generally leads to a fibrinous scar tissue, whereas a liver injury can result in complete liver regeneration. During the process of healing many of the early mediators are still needed, but also other mediators are getting involved. These include interleukins, lymphokines, chemokines and interferons — together referred to as cytokines. Many cell types contribute to the production of these cytokines at different stages during the entire track from the acute inflammation towards healing.

If the inflammation state continues to exist beyond two weeks, by definition, a chronic inflammation is in place. All the cellular and biochemical components are still in place and proceed with the inflammatory response as described for the acute inflammation. The situation is characterized by a dense infiltration of lymphocytes and macrophages. The body may be attempting to wall off and isolate the injury site through formation of a granuloma. Granulomas are often associated with the formation of multinucleated giant cells that form out of the fusion of a number of macrophages.

Healing can have several results. The tissue can be completely regenerated (resolution) or tissue can be repaired by cleaning (debridement) and subsequent scar tissue formation. Two phases are discerned during resolution and repair: the reconstructive and the maturation phases. The reconstructive phase takes up to two weeks and is characterized by fibroblast proliferation and collagen synthesis, epithelialization, and cellular differentiation. During this phase granulation tissue appears that is defined by the presence of new capillaries, fibroblasts and macrophages. The fibroblasts are responsible for the collagen synthesis and the resulting tissue reconstruction. The final maturation phase can take up to two years, with continuing differentiation of the cells, wound contraction, scar formation and scar remodeling.

Implanted Materials and Inflammation

Implanting a biomaterial in the body is largely comparable to wounding the body with a wood splinter. Largely, because the wood splinter creates an open wound with access to the outside world, allowing the entrance of microorganisms, whereas the biomaterial implantation occurs in a sterile operative theatre with peri-operative antimicrobial care. The response towards the wood splinter is well known to those who have experienced it. After a couple of weeks the splinter easily comes out of the wound in the presence of some kind of pus (exudate) and some weeks later the wound is entirely closed.

The body has effectively sealed of the surrounding tissue from the splinter by way of an epithelium layer around the splinter. The exudate represents the entire spectrum of invaded cells, proteins, cellular debris and killed microorganisms. And finally, the wound closure occurs due to the maturation phase of wound healing. Without proper measures a similar process will happen with percutaneous implants. These are devices that penetrate the skin on a continuous basis, thus increasing the risk of infection. Besides infection, the greatest risk for implant failure with these devices is the occurrence of marsupialization or extrusion, where the formation of a pocket or pouch continuous with the adjacent epithelial membrane ultimately pushes the implant outward.

The insertion of any implant in the body at any implantation site results in injury, as with every surgical procedure. The rules of inflammation/wound healing apply to this situation. A scheme of the healing process is shown in Fig. 2. With any implant there will be a stage where exudate infiltrates the tissue surrounding the implantation site. This is accompanied by the presence of neutrophilic granulocytes and, later on, macrophages. This stage is common to all implantations, but from here on several divergent pathways can be taken. In these pathways the normal stages of wound healing can be recognized.

The presence of the material often results in a chronic inflammation, by way of definition, if the inflammation goes on for more than two weeks. The chronic inflammation appearance in histological sections can be quite diverse, but contains macrophages, monocytes, lymphocytes, blood vessels and connective tissue. If the mononuclear cells (lymphocytes, plasma cells, macrophages) continue to be present, a true chronic inflammation occurs. On the other hand, if granulation tissue occurs, a normal wound healing response to implanted biomaterials is present. The granulation tissue can be initiated during both the acute and the chronic inflammatory response. Finally, the granulation tissue is transformed into either a fibrous capsule or a functional, regenerated tissue, depending on the site of implantation and the material/device characteristics. This is in accordance with the normal wound-healing response. Chronic inflammation, however, may also result in a foreign-body reaction. This reaction involves foreign-body giant cells (multinucleated giant cells) amid

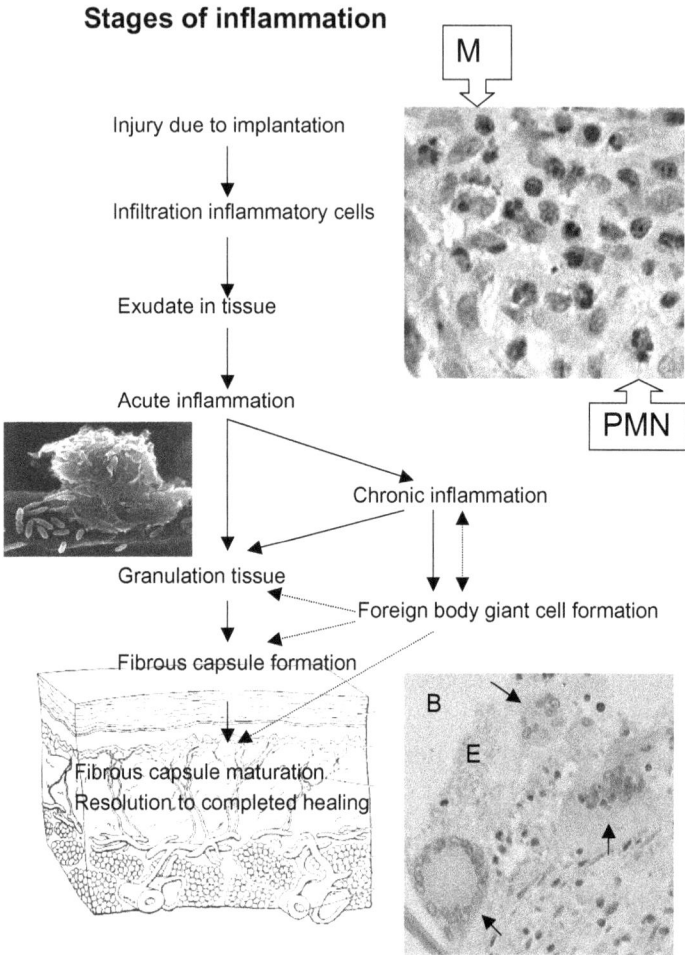

Fig. 2.   The stages of inflammation are schematically shown, including the key cellular players in the process, i.e. monocytes/macrophages (MØ), granulocytes (PMN) and foreign body giant cells (arrows). B = Biomaterial, E = Erythrocyte.

components of granulation tissue. The reaction can be present at the material interface for the lifetime of the implant. The foreign-body reaction directly apposing the implanted material can be walled off by the body by means of fibrous encapsulation.

For all permanent, non-degrading materials and devices the situation described above is valid. Many materials nowadays are degradable. During the process of degradation the tissues surrounding the implant are confronted with different situations. This can result in the appearance of stages of the wound-healing response in a random order and time kinetics, depending on the degradation products released at the implant site.

The ultimate tissue response to the presence of the material is part of the biocompatibility of this material. Biocompatibility refers to the capacity of a material to fulfill its function with an appropriate response for a specific application from the receiving host. An alternative definition is the quality of being accepted in a specific living environment without adverse or unwanted side effects. In this respect it is clear that the long-term presence of a chronic inflammatory response or foreign-body response is unwanted. In those situations implant materials generally are not considered to be biocompatible.

Soft Tissue Responses

In general, the stages of the wound-healing response are easily recognized in implantation procedures in the soft tissues, especially the subcutaneous pocket, as shown in Figs. 3 and 4. This is the most frequent implantation site in testing in animal models and therefore we focus on this implantation site. Other sites include the intramuscular and intraperitoneal sites. Organ-specific sites can also be used, such as the myocardial infarct site and lesion sites in liver, kidney and skin.

In subcutaneous implantations, a cut is made through the full thickness of the skin. Subsequently, a pocket is created directly underneath the skin by blunt dissection. The implant then is positioned in the pocket, and the wound is closed by placing stitches through the different layers of the skin. The entire procedure is simple and straightforward. During the surgical procedure, special attention is given to the fact that the surgery is performed under sterile conditions in order to avoid bacterial contamination of the wound site. In animals such as

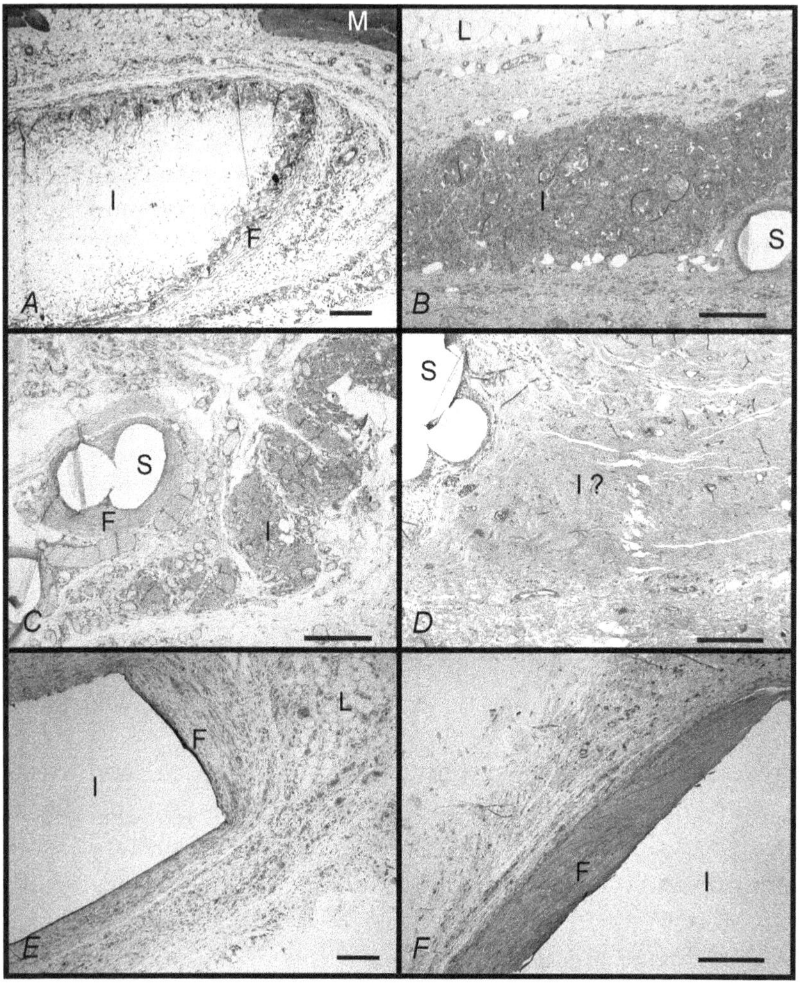

Fig. 3. Soft tissue response overview: A degradable, highly porous polyurethane was implanted subcutaneously and explanted at times of 4 (**A**), 26 (**B**), 52 (**C**) and 78 (**D**) weeks. The tissue ingrowth into the implant (I) is evident from week 4 to week 26. This is accompanied by implant material degradation and removal. The implant location was marked with a non-degradable suture (S) which is encapsulated with a fibrous capsule (F). After 78 weeks, virtually all material had disappeared with the ongoing process of resolution. In (**E**) and (**F**) the response to a non-degradable, non-porous polyethylene disc is shown after 4 weeks (**E**) and 52 weeks (**F**). A maturation of the fibrous capsule (F) is evident. L is adipose tissue, M is muscle tissue. Bars indicate 200 μm.

rabbits and rats, the usual subjects of implantation, the success rate for this kind of implantation procedure is high.

After implantation, the wound healing response is evaluated at time points ranging from one day to three years, depending on the type of material implanted. Often, researchers aim to map the entire kinetics of the wound healing response. Especially with degrading materials, a long follow-up time is often needed because the body has to deal with degradation products that are released over time. As described above, the response to inert materials leads to a matured tissue response within weeks after implantation, thus requiring only a short follow-up time.

Tissues initially will have similar responses to degradable and non-degradable materials. But as the tissue interacts with the degrading material interface and degradation products are released in the surrounding area, the responses start to differ from each other. This is exemplified in Fig. 3. From this figure, it is evident that inert materials are progressively surrounded by a fibrous capsule, without signs of the presence of inflammatory cells. Sometimes it is observed that inflammatory cells appear between the capsule and the inert material interface, in specific macrophages, but also granulocytes. In these cases, the inflammatory response continues over time, despite the presence of the capsular wall. This is an indication that the material is not truly biocompatible. The ongoing inflammation may be caused by products leaching out of the material, or by incompatible surface properties. From Fig. 4A it can be seen that a capsule is also formed around the degradable material. Despite the capsule, the scaffold material in invaded by connective tissue. Due to this invasion the fibrous capsule diminishes over time and finally disappears. During this time, foreign body giant cells are transiently present. Macrophages continue to be present as long as degradation fragments continue to appear. The macrophages take up these fragments and seem to take care of their further degradation. The connective tissue invasion of the degradable scaffolds is accompanied by the formation of capillaries and thus shows aspects of granulation tissue.

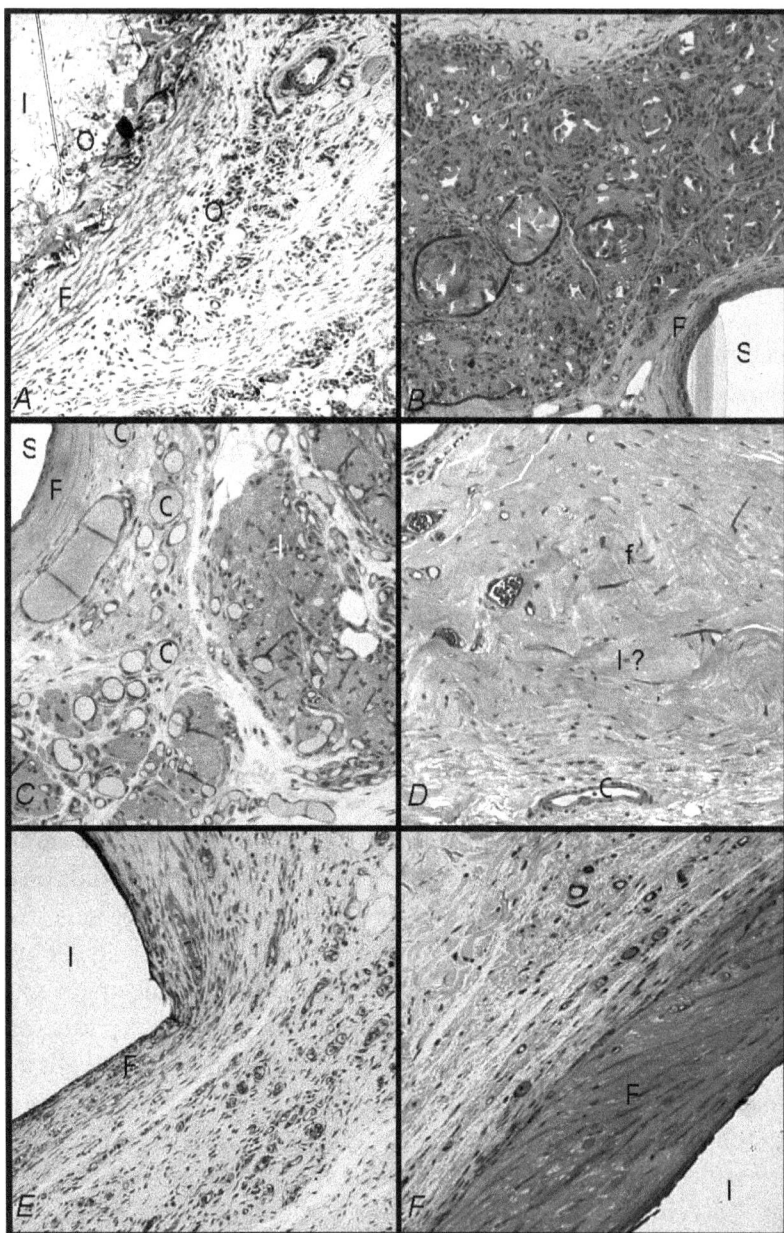

Fig. 4.   The soft-tissue response details of Fig. 3: (**A**)–(**F**) refer to the same materials and timepoints as shown in Fig. 3. O — Presence of inflammatory cells, F — Fibrous capsule, V — Vessel, I — Implant, S — Suture, C — Capillary, f — Fibroblasts.

The example given above illustrates the problems encountered in assessing the tissue response to implanted materials. Generally, the prolonged presence of inflammatory cells is considered to be an undesirable wound-healing response. As stated earlier, this response usually ends within two weeks, otherwise it becomes chronic. This is true for inert materials as shown in Fig. 3E/F. But for degrading materials, the situation is entirely different. With these materials, a chronic inflammation is fully acceptable as long as there will be a gradual decline when the degradation is completed. Furthermore, there should not be a sudden burst of released degradation products that cannot be handled by the surrounding tissues. Another potential danger is that some degradation products accumulate in tissues or macrophages without further degradation. These products can be responsible for inflammatory reactions years after implantation.

Hard Tissue Responses

For biomaterials implanted in "hard" tissues, such as bone, cartilage and teeth, in general the same principles apply as for biomaterials in soft tissues. However, there are some special issues to address. In general, the body will recognize the implant as a foreign body, and will try to eliminate the intruder. The first step in this process is the isolation of the implant by surrounding it with a capsule. Vascularization of the capsule provides the ways for the cells of the body's defense system to enter the capsule and try to degrade the implanted material. The amount of capsule formed depends on the reactivity of the material implanted (inertness) and whether the material is recognized as foreign body. Some materials used as implants in bone and

---

In (A) and (B) it is evident that many inflammatory cells, predominantly macrophages, are involved in the tissue response. These cells arrive at the edge of the implant and subsequently start to invade the porous implant. Initially, a fibrous capsule is formed (A), but inflammatory cells are already present at the implant side. The invasion of cells/tissue is accompanied by the presence of capillaries (granulation tissue) that become very pronounced in stage C. Note that both the sutures and the polyethylene show a maturing fibrous capsule without the presence of significant amounts of inflammatory cells.

teeth are not recognized by the body as "foreign," and are not encapsulated. This applies for the calcium phosphate ceramics and bioglasses, which very much resemble the minerals naturally occurring in these tissues, but also some polymers as shown in Fig. 5.

Calcium phosphate ceramics are considered to be osteoconductive. Osteoconductivity implies the ability of a substance to support the attachment and migration of osteogenic cells, either osteoblasts or osteo-progenitor cells from the wound. Furthermore, most calcium phosphate ceramics also support osteogenic differentiation of osteo-progenitor cells. The molecular mechanisms by which these events occur are not fully understood. High local concentrations of calcium and phosphate ions, which are assumed to be present, have been proposed to be responsible for these phenomena. A major disadvantage of calcium phosphate ceramics is their brittleness, which makes the use of these materials less suitable for filling large bone defects.

Calcium Phosphate Coatings

When calcium phosphates are used as coating for metal implants, as is done with all kinds of endoprostheses, the coating serves two purposes: first, the coating provides a substrate for good bone bonding; and second the coating prevents the formation of a connective tissue membrane (capsule) around the metal implant at the sites which are coated.

Calcium phosphate coatings of metal implants are applied by a process called scintering. Calcium phosphate is sprayed on the implant in high temperature flames. This process results in highly crystalline calcium phosphates, which are biocompatible, but also difficult to degrade by osteoclasts.

Recently, the principles of biomimetics have resulted in the preparation of amorphous calcium phosphate coatings of different kinds at physiological temperatures. Biomimetic calcium phosphate coatings also are not recognized as foreign bodies and are excellent substrates for osteoblasts and bone deposition. Preparation of these coatings at physiological temperature allows incorporation of proteins, vitamins or even cells in or on the coating. A biomimetic

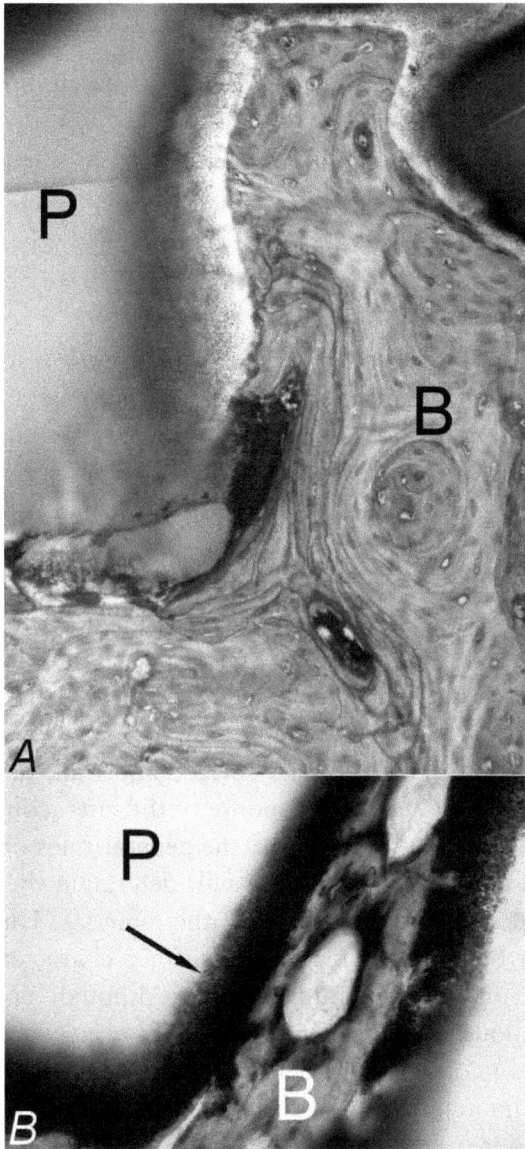

Fig. 5. Implanted 1000 60/40 PEOT/PBT polymer in a bone defect in a rabbit femur (Methylene Blue and basic fuchsin staining, original magnification 100 ×). (**A**). The bone (B) is firmly attached to the polymer (P). (**B**). Detail (von Kossa staining, original magnification 400 ×) illustrating calcium phosphate crystals on the surfaces of the polymer (arrow) to which the bone is attached (See also Bouwmeester *et al.*, (1998) *J Mater Sci* 9:181–189).

octa-calcium phosphate coating with incorporated bone morpho-genetic protein-2 (BMP2) has been shown to be a slow-release drug delivery system. Subcutaneous implantation of titanium discs with this coating results in ectopic bone formation, which makes these coatings osteoinductive. Biomimetic calcium phosphates are more easily resorbed compared to sintered calcium phosphates.

Concluding Remarks

Material surfaces have been shown to influence the response of cells interacting with these surfaces. The surface's atomic and molecular composition, the charge distribution and the overall wettability determine parameters of cell behavior such as adhesion, spreading, proliferation and function. These interactions are mainly mediated by biological macromolecules within the conditioning film, which can actively be modified by the interacting cells. A better understanding of the modular design, as well as the diverse functions of these macromolecules, has led to the development of material surface modifications with incorporated biological elements or their mimics, such as adhesion peptides and growth and differentiation factors. As a result, an increasing number of material surface and bulk designs appear that can modulate or steer the response of the interacting cells.

Upon implantation in the body, the general rules of the wound-healing reaction, i.e. inflammation, will determine the outcome of the tissue response to the presence of the material. The outcome is dependent on both the bulk and the surface characteristics of the material and on the implantation site. Although not enough is known yet about how designed material surface properties will influence the outcome, it is evident that a rational use of these properties will ultimately allow us to tune the wound healing reaction according to our needs.

References — General Reading

Ratner BD, Hoffman AS, Schoen FJ, Lemons JE (eds.). (2004) *Biomaterials Science: An Introduction to Materials in Medicine*, 2nd ed. Elsevier Academic Press.

Probing cell-material surface interactions

1. Schoen FJ, Mitchell RN. (2004) Tissues, the extracellular matrix, and cell-biomaterial interactions. In: Ratner BD, Hoffman AS, Schoen FJ, Lemons JE (eds.), *Biomaterials Science: An Introduction to Materials in Medicine*, 2nd ed. Elsevier Academic Press, Chapter 3.4, 260–82.

Material surface composition

1. Castner DG, Ratner BD. (2002) Biomedical surface science: foundations to frontiers. *Surf Sci* 500:28–60.
2. Hutmacher DW, Garcia AJ. (2005) Scaffold-based bone engineering by using genetically modified cells. *Gene* 347:1–10.

The role of the extracellular matrix

1. Lutolf MP, Hubbell JA. (2005) Synthetic biomaterials as instructive extracellular microenvironments for morphogenesis in tissue engineering. *Nature Biotech* 23:47–55.
2. Garcia AJ. (2005) Get a grip: integrins in cell–biomaterial interactions. *Biomaterials* 26:7525–9.
3. Wilson CJ, Clegg RE, Leavesley DI, Pearcy MJ. (2005) Mediation of biomaterial-cell interactions by adsorbed proteins: a review. *Tiss Eng* 11:1–18.

Inflammation is a fundamental response of the body towards injury

1. McCance & Huether. (2002) Pathophysiology. The Biological Basis for Disease in Adults and Children, 4th ed., pp. 197–221.

Implanted materials and inflammation

1. Anderson JM. (2004) Inflammation, wound healing, and the foreign-body response. In: Ratner BD, Hoffman AS, Schoen FJ, Lemons JE (eds.), *Biomaterials Science: An Introduction to Materials in Medicine*, 2nd ed. Elsevier Academic Press, Chapter 4.2, pp. 296–304.

Soft tissue responses

1. Cadee JA, van Luyn MJA, Brouwer LA, *et al.* (2000) *In vivo* biocompatibility of dextran-based hydrogels. *Biomed Mater Res* 50:397–404.
2. Parker JA, Walboomers XF, von den Hoff JW, *et al.* (2002) Soft-tissue response to silicone and poly-L-lactic acid implants with a periodic or random surface micropattern. *J Biomed Mater Res* 61(1):91–8.
3. Parker JA, Walboomers XF, von den Hoff HJ, *et al.* (2002) Soft tissue response to microtextured silicone and poly-L-lactic acid implants: fibronectin pre-coating vs. radio-frequency glow discharge treatment. *Biomaterials* 23:3545–53.

4. Parker JA, Walboomers XF, von den Hoff JW, *et al.* (2002) The effect of bone anchoring and micro-grooves on the soft tissue reaction to implants. *Biomaterials* 23:3887–96.
5. van Minnen B, van Leeuwen MBM, Stegenga B, *et al.* (2005) Short-term *in vitro* and *in vivo* biocompatibility of a biodegradable polyurethane foam based on 1,4-butanediisocyanate. *J Mat Sci Mat Med* 16:221–7.

Hard tissue responses

1. Barrere F, Layrolle P. (1999) Physical and chemical characteristics of plasma-sprayed and biomimetic apatite coating. *Bioceramics* 12:125–8.
2. Barrere F, Layrolle P. (2001) Biomimetic coatings on titanium: a crystal growth study of octacalcium phosphate. *J Mater Sci Mater Med* 12(6):529–34.
3. Barrere F, Layrolle P, van Blitterswijk CA, de Groot K. (1999) Biomimetic calcium phosphate coatings on Ti6AI4V: a crystal growth study of octacalcium phosphate and inhibition by $Mg2+$ and $HCO3$. *Bone* 25(2):107S–111S.
4. Barrere F, Van Der Valk CM, Dalmeijer RA, *et al.* (2003) Osteogenicity of octacalcium phosphate coatings applied on porous metal implants. *J Biomed Mater Res* 66A(4):779–88.
5. Geesink RGT. (2002) Osteoconductive coatings for total hip arthroplasty. *Clin Orthop* 395:53–65.
6. Habibovic P, Barrere F. (2002) Biomimetic hydroxyapatite coating on metal implants. *Am Ceram Soc* 85(3):517–22.
7. Liu Y, de Groot K, Hunziker EB. (2005) BMP-2 liberated from biomimetic implant coatings induces and sustains direct ossification in an ectopic rat model. *Bone* 36(5):745–57.
8. Liu Y, Hunziker EB, Layrolle P, *et al.* (2004) Bone morphogenetic protein 2 incorporated into biomimetic coatings retains its biological activity. *Tiss Eng* 10(1–2):101–8.

Chapter 7

Biomaterial-associated Surgery and Infection — A Review of the Literature

P.G.M. Maathuis*, S.K. Bulstra*, H.C. van der Mei[†],
J.R. van Horn[‡] and H.J. Busscher[†]

The incidence of wound infection after clean surgery is often underestimated. Infection rates up to 15% can be found by meticulous follow up. The consequences of these infectious complications can be troublesome for the patient involved. Most of the time the post-operative recovery will be delayed and secondary healing of the operative wound will occur. The long-term consequences of these infectious complications will be within acceptable limits. However, when biomaterials are involved in post-operative infectious complications, a totally different scenario is likely to occur — the longevity of these artificial organs and temporary assist devices is limited by biomaterial-associated infection of the implant.

*Department of Orthopedics, University Medical Center Groningen, Hanzeplein 1, 9713 GZ Groningen, The Netherlands.
[†]Department of BioMedical Engineering, University Medical Center Groningen, A. Deusinglaan 1, 9713 AV Groningen, The Netherlands.
[‡]Department of Orthopedics, University Medical Center Groningen, Groningen, The Netherlands, address: Wageningse Berg 104, 3524 LS Utrecht, The Netherlands.

119

In this chapter we present an overview of the mechanisms of biomaterial-associated infection and its occurrence in various medical disciplines. Surgical procedures are critically reviewed for non-biomaterial associated versus biomaterial-associated surgery and recommendations are given for biomaterial-associated surgery.

Introduction

The incidence of wound infection after clean surgery is often underestimated. Infection rates up to 15% can be found by meticulous follow up.[1] The consequences of these infectious complications can be troublesome for the patient involved. Most of the time the post-operative recovery will be delayed and secondary healing of the operative wound will occur. The long-term consequences of these infectious complications will be within acceptable limits. However, when biomaterials are involved in post-operative infectious complications, a totally different scenario is likely to occur — the longevity of these artificial organs and temporary assist devices is limited by biomaterial-associated infection of the implant. Biomaterial-associated infections are usually resistant to antibiotics. Removal of an infected implant is the final outcome of most of these infections, at high costs for the health care system and discomfort for the patient. Ever since the description by Gristina of biomaterial-associated infection as "a race for the surface"[2,3] between microbial adhesion and tissue integration, there is a growing awareness of the risk of foreign body implantation. The design of a biomaterial surface upon which the race for the surface is fought determines the outcome of it, as it depends upon a delicate fine-tuning of the properties of the biomaterial surface that has not yet been achieved.

Some infected biomaterial implants are relatively easily removed, like contact lenses,[4] voice prostheses[5] or dentures.[6] The total artificial heart,[7] elongatable endoprostheses as used after extensive tumor resection in children, and total hip and knee prostheses, on the other hand, are much more difficult to remove. Moreover, removal of these devices often constitutes a clinical dilemma; for instance, the removal of an infected Hickmann catheter in patients on chemotherapeutic treatment. Here the surgeon has to choose between two evils: leaving the infected catheter in place or removal at the expense of stopping the chemotherapy (note that a new catheter can only be safely inserted once the infection has fully cleared, otherwise recurrence will happen in due time). Biomaterial implants sometimes are complex devices made of a combination of different biomaterials. These materials need to be compatible with their biological environment, which is not always the first concern of the biomedical engineer, as mechanical and manufacturing properties often dictate the choice for a given material. Tables 1 and 2 list commonly used biomedical implants in modern medicine with their incidence of clinical infectious problems.

> Completely sterile surgery is impossible.

Different biomaterials are prone to infection by different organisms. *Staphylococcus aureus* is generally found on metallic implants,[25] while pseudomonas and *Staphylococcus epidermidis* are mainly isolated from polymeric implants.[25,26] Consequently, as more different biomaterials are involved in an implant, this increases the chance of a biomaterial-associated infection and the recognition of strains being pathogenic. *S. epidermidis* was long considered non-pathogenic and harmless member of the normal skin microflora, but only became a pathogen in the era of biomaterial implants.

Table 1. Incidences of Infection of Different Biomedical Devices in Permanent Contact with Skin and/or Outer Human Body Environment

Body Site	Implant or Device	Incidence of Infectious Complications Necessitating Exchange
Urethra	Foley catheter	2.79/1000 catheter days[8]
Venous system	Peripheral inserted Central Venous catheters	2–5/1000 catheter days[9]
Arterial system	Arterial catheters	0.4–0.7%[10]
Intraperitoneal	Peritoneal dialysis catheters	11–13%[101]
Extremities	Pins in external fracture fixation	12–71%[12]
Oral cavity	Dental implants	5–10%[13]
Laryngeal cavity	Voice prosthesis	Every 4 months[14]

Table 2. Incidence of Infection of Different Biomedical Implants Arranged According to Body Site

Body Site	Implant or Device	Incidence of Infection
Subcutaneous	Cardiac pacemaker	1–5%[15]
	Tissue expanders	0.9%[16]
	Chin augmentation implants	0.8%[17]
Soft tissue	Mammary prosthesis	2–2.5%[18]
	Abdominal wall patches	3–8%[19]
	Penile prostheses	2–10%[20]
	Nasal implants	3.2%[21]
	Intraocular lenses	0.49%[22]
Circulatory system	Prosthetic heart valve	1–3%[13]
	Dacron aortoiliofemoral bypasses	2–10%[23]
Bone	Total hip prosthesis	1%[24]
	Total knee prosthesis	2%[24]

Surgery is supposed to be done in a sterile way, but it can easily be argued that completely sterile surgery is impossible. In a contamination study of primary total hip arthroplasties, 30% of the materials in contact with the prosthesis site harvested viable micro-organisms.[27] Nearly the same percentage was found by Knobben *et al.* in two different studies.[28,29]

Troublesome in biomaterial-associated infections is the long history of antibiotic therapy applied prior to the ultimate decision to remove the implant, giving the opportunity for antibiotic resistance to develop. Van de Belt *et al.*[30] described the culturing of antibiotic-resistant staphylococci from gentamicin-loaded bone cement that was removed in a hip revision for infection. The path of entry of infecting micro-organisms to a biomaterial implant can be directly along the parts of the implant itself, like along the polyvinylchloride drive lines of the total artificial heart[38] or through haematogenous spreading[31] or dental treatment.[32] Alternatively, it can be stated that, despite the use of intra-operative systemic antibiotic prophylactics, strict hygienic protocols, sterile operating theatres and special sterile enclosure, prostheses almost inevitably become contaminated during surgery and will be implanted in this state. Subsequently, whether or not clinical signs of infection develop depends on an interplay of the host immune system and the microbiological characteristics of the infecting organisms.

In this chapter we present an overview of the mechanisms of biomaterial-associated infection and its occurrence in various medical disciplines. Surgical procedures are critically reviewed for non-biomaterial associated versus biomaterial-associated surgery and recommendations are given for biomaterial-associated surgery.

The "Race for the Surface" and Biofilm Formation

Several authors have proposed a model for biofilm formation in general,[33,34] which has been developed to the concept of "the race for the surface," as first formulated by Gristina in 1987.[2]

Micro-organisms have a strong tendency to become attached to surfaces. On these surfaces they form a micro-ecosystem in which different microbial strains and species grow in a slime-enclosed biofilm. Biofilm formation involves a sequence of events,[33,34] represented in Fig. 1. The first step is the adsorption of small, macromolecular components that form a so-called "conditioning film" on the surface of the biomaterial involved. The formation of this conditioning film is extremely fast and occurs in seconds after exposure to a biological environment. The biological environment in which the biomaterial is placed determines the nature of the adsorbed macromolecules. For instance, dental restorative materials adsorb salivary proteins, contact lenses adsorb proteins and lipid components from tear fluid, while blood contacting biomaterials adsorb a variety of different plasma proteins prior to the arrival of the first micro-organism. A prerequisite for microbial adhesion to occur is an adsorbed conditioning film, which changes the physico-chemical properties of the interacting surfaces. Adherence of micro-organisms on bare biomaterials surfaces is rare.

The initial adhesion of micro-organisms is reversible and depends on the overall physico-chemical characteristics of the microbial cell surface, the biomaterials surface and the biological bathing fluid.

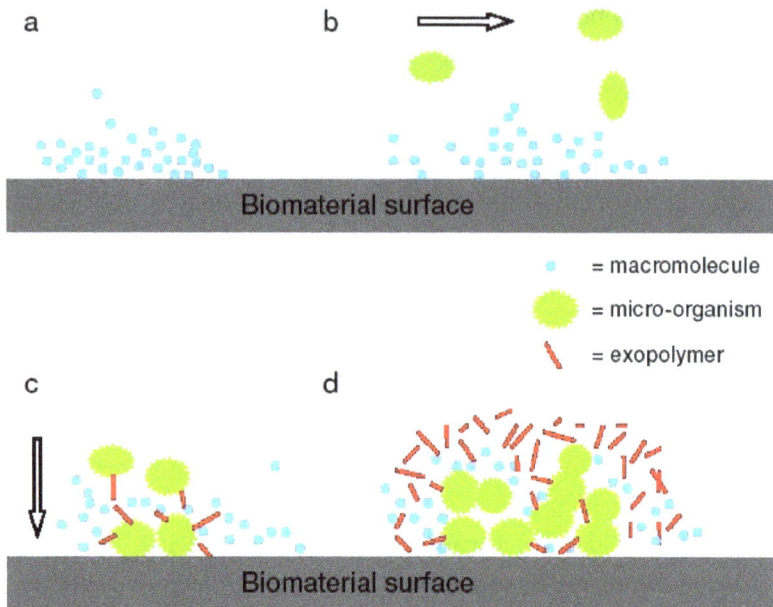

Fig. 1. Sequential steps in the formation of biofilms on a biomaterial surface, including:
- Formation of a conditioning film
- Microbial mass transport
- Initial microbial adhesion and anchoring through exopolymer production
- Growth of adhering micro-organisms

Reprinted with permission of H. van de Belt.

Firm anchoring through exopolymer production may change this reversible adhesion to an irreversible state. The exopolymers surrounding the micro-organisms embed the biofilm to form the so-called "glycocalix."[35]

In addition to anchoring, the glycocalix offers protection against environmental attacks and antibiotics.[36–38] Multiplication of the adhering organisms is the main mechanism of growth in a biofilm and eventually leads to the formation of a thick film. The growth rate due to a lowered metabolism is generally slowed down in the biofilm as compared with a planktonic state of growth. Because of this lowered state of metabolism, the sensitivity for certain antibiotics is reduced. Also, bacteria in this quiescent state are hard to detect with standard microbiologic techniques. This puts the concept of "aseptic loosening" in, for example, orthopaedic implant surgery in another perspective, as will be discussed later.

In the final phase of biofilm formation, organisms on the periphery of the expanding biofilm may detach or disaggregate, which plays an important role in the pathogenesis of septic processes.

Biomaterials and Microorganisms

The host defence is significantly compromised in the presence of a foreign material.[39] In continuation of this concept, the resistance of osteomyelitis and foreign body-related infections to antibiotic therapy was rationalized by others.[40,41] Furthermore, the relatively avirulent *S. epidermidis*, normally not capable of establishing infection, has become the most common causative organism in biomaterial-associated infection.[42]

The organisms causing a biomaterial-associated infection may have one or more of several possible sources. The first source is constituted by the skin. During insertion of the biomaterial, micro-organisms from the skin can be pushed towards the implant surface. A second source is constituted by airborne micro-organisms, which, in varying concentrations, are normally present in the operating theatre. They can reach the surface as early as before implantation.[43,44] A third source described is the haematogenous spread of micro-organisms from distant foci in the body towards the biomaterial site. Anecdotal reports of sepsis following dental work and other bacteraemia-producing procedures like surgical incision of infectious processes are common. However, well-documented accounts on this subject are rare.[45,31]

Biomaterial-implants in permanent contact with skin and/or the outer human body environment form a class of implants that have, by definition, a contamination rate of 100%. This contaminated state makes them very susceptible to malfunction because of infectious complications (see Table 1).[46] Clinical examples of these biomaterial-implants are intravenous catheters, peritoneal dialysis catheters, urinary tract catheters, voice prostheses, oral implants and percutaneous pins in external fracture fixation. Lower infection rates have been observed with totally implanted prostheses (see Fig. 2), the consequences being more serious, though.

Surgical Precautions and Consequences

Because implants in permanent contact with skin and/or the outer human body environment have a 100% contamination rate, they have a high chance of malfunction due to infectious complications. Therefore, besides the regular surgical precautions, preventive measures are being developed. This is exemplified by the coating with silver of percutaneous catheters[47,11] and percutaneous pins.[48] In the field of preventing infection of percutaneous pins, the use of a small electric current has proved to be effective in animal experiments.[49]

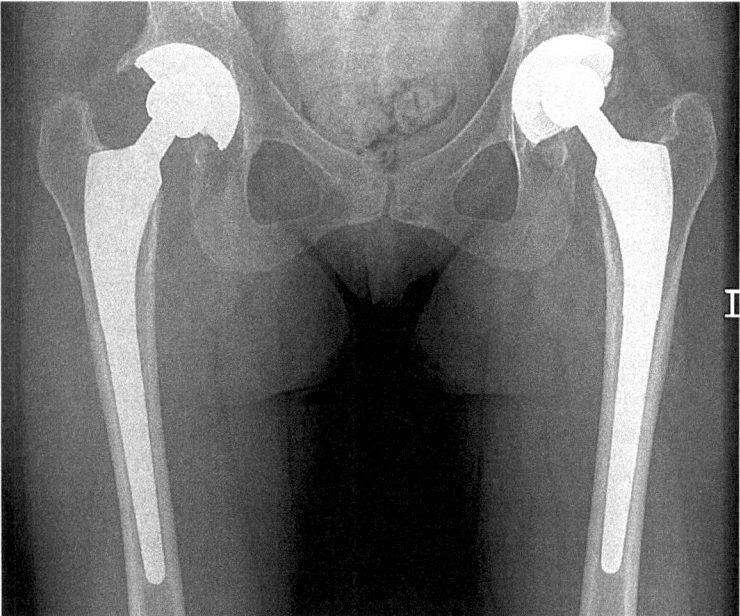

Fig. 2.   Roentgenographic example of patient with uncemented total hip prostheses implanted on both sides.

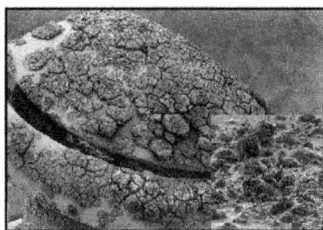

Fig. 3.   Example of a voice prosthesis covered with biofilm, causing a malfunction in the valve mechanism.

The consequences of the development of a microbial biofilm can be impairment of the function of the implant or device and/or worsening of the clinical state of the patient. Because microorganisms block the valve mechanism, a proper functioning of the voice prosthesis (see Fig. 3) is impaired or causes leakage of food into the trachea.[50] An exchange procedure every four months of the prosthesis is the result of this process.[14] Colonization by microorganisms of urinary tract catheters is inevitable. This can cause blockage or, more seriously, bacteriuria.[51] Infections of indwelling catheters, such as, for example, central venous catheters, often results in bacteraemia, which can cause sepsis and endocarditis. With infections of implants in the circulatory system, a high mortality rate of 50% and 70% occurs for vascular grafts and prosthetic valves, respectively.[52]

Infection of deep tissue implants, for example, orthopaedic implants, will usually result in serious complications like pain, swelling of the joint or limb, and loosening of the implant. Mortality rates up to 20% are reported with these kind of implants.[53-55] Up to a year after microbial seeding, clinical signs of deep implant infections are being reported to appear.[56]

This long interval between inoculation of the bacteria and the onset of symptoms can be caused by the low-virulence organisms which normally inhabit the skin and oral cavity. This may often mimic the natural "aseptic" loosening of prostheses.[57,58] Because of this low-virulence character of the organisms involved, in combination with the biofilm they grow in, a significant part of these infections is probably never recognized. As standard microbiological techniques are used to test the presence of infectious micro-organisms, slow-growing biofilm organisms often remain undetected.[59-61]

This has important clinical implications for the concept of "aseptic loosening" and the recurrent nature of musculoskeletal infection. Nelson *et al.*[62] explained this with a sort of triple mechanism, including (1) inadequate techniques of removing adherent, biofilm-associated bacteria; (2) small colony-forming variants; and (3) intracellular *S. aureus* "residing" within osteoclasts.

> The main goal of a biomaterial-associated surgery protocol is decreasing contamination by minimization of air disturbance.

Generally speaking a surgeon needs to perform his surgical technique well with regard not only to placing the incision, soft tissue handling, meticulous haemostasis and operating time, but also with regard to such simple things as the application of the correct time of scrubbing hands, proper use of hair and mouth covers and the maintenance of a strict discipline in the operating theatre. The latter aspects are most important in biomaterial-associated surgery, and because of their relative unimportance in soft tissue surgery, are frequently overlooked in implant surgery. One must realize that the most common cause of biomaterial-associated infection is thought to be peri-operative contamination.[63]

Avoidance of devitalization by meticulous handling of tissue is an important variable in influencing the risks of deep infection. To prevent areas of skin necrosis between an old and a new incision, previous incisions should be used. Local factors such as scar tissue, depending on its size and localization, can have a decreased vascularity and it may greatly increase the time required to perform revision surgery.[43,64,65] Especially when infection has been the reason for earlier operations, the outcome can be adversely affected.[66,67] Meticulous haemostasis and wound closure are essential in preventing haematoma or an area of wound necrosis. Operative time has to be kept to a minimum because of the association of operative time and the development of infection.[43]

Biomaterial-associated Surgery versus Non-Biomaterial Associated Surgery

The incidence of infection after implant surgery is generally low (see Table 2) and infection rates have decreased substantially over the past decades, but the often disastrous results of these infections make them important complications. Also, because of the increasing incidence of, for example, total joint replacement, infection still is a source of considerable morbidity.[68]

Apart from the morbidity, the financial burden a joint prosthesis infection puts on health care systems is enormous. In the United States the annual cost to treat the 3,500 to 4,000 infections that develop after arthroplasties each year is between US$150 and US$200 million.[69] In spinal surgery the use of spinal instrumentation clearly increases the risk for post-operative infection from 1% to a range of 2.1% to 8.5%.[70] A large amount of the US$24 billion spent in 1990 on treating spinal disorders[71] will therefore account for the cost of treating spinal implant infections in the near future. With an increasing use of biomaterials in surgery, this financial problem will only continue to increase.

It can be argued that sterile implantation of biomaterials is impossible. The operation wound is contaminated to some extent in all procedures. Minimizing contamination by optimizing the operating-room environment, protocols and the operative technique is crucial. These are the factors that can be influenced by the surgeon and the operating personnel. Performing biomaterial-associated surgery means being aware of the possibilities of contamination during the procedure. This necessitates an Operating Room (OR) discipline in operating personnel, as well as in anesthetists, nurses, students, porters and visitors who enter the aseptic zone.

When a surgeon implants biomaterials, an important compromising factor concerning the host defense is introduced. In a classical study in humans it was shown that the presence of a subcutaneous suture reduced the required inoculum to produce infection with *S. aureus* from 10[6] to only 200 bacteria.[39] Thus, the presence of a foreign body presents another clinical challenge on its own.

Whenever a biomaterial is introduced into the human body, surgical and mechanical trauma, as well as the biomaterial itself will evoke an acute inflammatory response.[72] This acute inflammatory cascade results in localized cell necrosis and tissue degeneration and the formation of a very thin membrane between the prosthesis and the body, consisting of fibroblasts, vascular endothelium cells and macrophages. This immune response can disappear when the wound is healed and the biomaterial is encapsulated. In many cases however the host-biomaterials interface remains in a state of chronic inflammation, as few metals and plastics are completely chemically inert in the warm, wet and oxygenated environment of living tissues with a non-neutral pH, causing the release of components of the biomaterial, like corrosion products, plasticizers and monomers which are able to incite an inflammatory reaction.[73,2] Chronic inflammation impairs host cell growth on the implant[74] and can cause chronic pain, while it may disrupt the anchorage of the implant into the surrounding tissues, thus impairing its stability and leading to failing performance.

Historically, orthopaedic surgeons are used to working with biomaterial implants on a large scale since the development of joint arthroplasties in the 1960s. Because they are familiar with the susceptibility of traumatized bone to infection, as has been shown in animal models of osteomyelitis,[75,76] their OR manners and attitude towards minimizing contamination have since then been further developed and fine-tuned. Charnley already initiated this after concluding that his 7% post-operative infection rate with total hip arthroplasty was too high and operative protocols needed to be updated.[43] Contamination of the operative wound is influenced by the OR environment. Variables affecting the OR hygienic efficiency include the number of people inside[77] and their adherence to adequate protocols[15,78]; the amount of traffic in the OR[77] and personnel present[10]; the preparation of the operative site[79,80]; the timing and technique of preoperative shaving[81]; and the clothing of the operating personnel,[82-84] including double-gloving, because of the chance of perforation[85] and contamination.[86] Although there seems to be consensus on the importance of a clean air environment in the OR, the role of laminar airflow in decreasing infection has remained controversial.[87,44] Some report an improvement in direct infection control[43,88-90] or indirect control by diminishing the prevalence of contamination of the surgical instruments.[91] Others report the influence of airflow on infection rates to be less important[92] or to be proven.[93]

Although the above-mentioned potential measures are important, the single most important variable influencing the development of post-operative implant infection is the appropriate use of peri-operative antibiotics.[92,94-96] Peri-operative antibiotics in implant surgery are now common practice.[97,98] The type of preferred antibiotic and its appropriate regimen has been studied by Tang *et al.*[99]

In addition, recording of the number of infections with feedback to the treating physician[100] should be integrated into a registration of complications in the department, as part of a continuous education program. This recording should preferably extend also to personnel in operating rooms and bacteriological and sterilization departments.[103]

Biomaterial-associated Surgery Protocol

Reducing biomaterial-associated infections in surgery involves a change in the operating attitude of everyone involved in all processes that are ongoing in the OR towards decreasing contamination risks. The non-biomaterial associated surgeon is used to a more forgiving environment where therapy-resistant infections are rare. Biomaterial-associated surgery by surgeons not familiar with the contamination risks and the ways of preventing them can be hazardous. To minimize these complications, the awareness of these contamination risks should be reflected in an appropriate protocol, adjusting of the peri-operative protocols, and attitude of the surgeon and operating personnel.

The exact content of such a protocol is hard to ascertain, because many statements are open for debate. Looking at the essentials, however, the main goal is decreasing contamination by minimization of air disturbance. Principles for achieving this goal in a biomaterial-associated surgery protocol are the minimizing of: personnel traffic in and out of the OR; personnel movement within the OR; and personnel communication.

Strict obedience by all those involved and continuous education through performance feedback, together with an appropriate antibiotic prophylaxis regime should minimize the inevitable post-operative infectious complications, with their devastating effect on the function and lifetime of the biomaterials involved, as well as on the patient who is the victim.

References

1. Leaper DJ, Melling AG. (2001) Antibiotic prophylaxis in clean surgery: clean non-implant wounds. *J Chemother* 1:96–101.
2. Gristina AG. (1987) Biomaterial-centered infection; microbial adhesion versus tissue integration. *Science* 237:1588–95.
3. Gristina AG, Naylor P, Myrvik Q. (1988) Infections from biomaterials and implants: a race for the surface. *Medical Progress through Technology* 14: 205–24.
4. Liesegang TJ. (1997) Contact lens related microbial keratitis: Part I: Epidemiology. *Cornea* 16:125–31.
5. Ackerstaff AH, Hilgers FJM, Meeuwis CA, *et al.* (1999) Multi-institutional assessment of the Provox 2 voice prostheses. *Arch Otolaryngol Head Neck Surg* 125:167–73.
6. Radford DR, Challacombe SJ, Walter JD. (1999) Denture plaque and adherence of *Candida albicans* to denture-base materials *in vivo* and *in vitro*. *Crit Rev Oral Biol Med* 10:99–116.
7. Gristina AG, Dobbins JJ, Giammara B, *et al.* (1988) Biomaterial-centered sepsis and the total artificial heart — microbial adhesion vs tissue integration. *JAMA* 259:870–4.
8. Luehm D, Fauerbach L. (1999) Task force studies. Infection rates, surgical site management and Foley catheter infections. *Caring* 18:30–4.
9. Safdar N, Maki DG. (2005) Risk of catheter-related bloodstream infection with peripherally inserted central venous catheters used in hospitalized patients. *Chest* 2:489–95.
10. Frezza EE, Mezghebe H. (1998) Indications and complications of arterial catheter use in surgical or medical intensive care units: analysis of 4932 patients. *Am Surg* 2:127–31.

11. Tobin EJ, Bambauer R. (2003) Silver coating of dialysis catheters to reduce bacterial colonization and infection. *Ther Apher Dial* 6:504–9.
12. Bernardo LM. (2001) Evidence-based practice for pin site care in injured children. *Orthop Nurs* 5:29–34.
13. Ehrlich GD, Stoodley P, Kathju S, *et al.* (2005) Engineering approaches for the detection and control of orthopaedic biofilm infections. *Clin Orthop* 437:59–66.
14. Van den Hoogen FA, Oudes MJ, Hombergen G, *et al.* (1996) The Groningen, Nijdam and Provox voice prostheses: a prospective clinical comparison based on 845 replacements. *Acta Otolaryngol* 116:119–24.
15. Borer A, Gilad J, Hyam E, *et al.* (2004) Prevention of infections associated with permanent cardiac antiarrhythmic devices by implementation of a comprehensive control program. *Infect Control Hosp Epidemiol* 6:492–7.
16. Disa JJ, Ad-El DD, Cohen SM, *et al.* (1999) The premature removal of tissue expanders in breast reconstruction. *Plast Reconstr Surg* 104:1662–5.
17. Gross EJ, Hamilton MM, Ackermann K, Perkins SW. (1999) Mersilene mesh chin augmentation. A 14-year experience. *Arch Facial Plast Surg* 1: 183–9.
18. Pittet B, Montandon D, Pittet D. (2005) Infection in breast implants. *Lancet Infect Dis* 5:94–106.
19. Deysine M. (1998) Pathophysiology, prevention, and management of prosthetic infections in hernia surgery. *Surg Clin North Am* 78:1105–15.
20. Schoepen Y, Staerman F. (2002) Penile prostheses and infection. *Prog Urol* 3:377–83.
21. Godin MS, Waldman SR, Johnson CM. (1999) Nasal augmentation using Gore-Tex. A 10-year experience. *Arch Facial Plast Surg* 1:118–21.
22. Khan RI, Kennedy S, Barry P. (2005) Incidence of presumed postoperative endophthalmitis in Dublin for a 5-year period (1997–2001). *J Cataract Refractive Surg* 31:1575–81.
23. Andreev, A. (1995) A 10-year follow-up study of bypass operations with double-velour dacron in the aortoiliofemoral position. *Khirurgiia Sofiia* 48:17–22.
24. Zimmerli W, Trampuz A, Ochsner PE. (2004) Prosthetic-joint infections. *N Engl J Med* 351:1645–54.
25. Barth E, Myrvik QM, Wagner W, Gristina AG. (1989) *In vitro* and *in vivo* comparative colonization of *Staphylococcus aureus* and *Staphylococus epidermidis* on orthopaedic implant materials. *Biomaterials* 10:325–8.
26. Ferreiros CM, Carballo J, Criado MT, *et al.* (1989) Surface free energy and interaction of *Staphylococcus epidermidis* with biomaterials. *FEMS Microbiol Lett* 51:89–94.
27. Maathuis PGM, Neut D, Busscher HJ, *et al.* (2005) Perioperative contamination in primary total hip arthroplasty. *Clin Orthop* 433:136–9.

28. Knobben BAS, Van Horn JR, Van der Mei HC, Busscher HJ. (2006, In press) Evaluation of measures to decrease intra-operative bacterial contamination in orthopaedic implant surgery. *J Hosp Infect.*

29. Knobben BAS, Engelsma Y, Neut D, *et al.* (2006, In press) Intra-operative contamination influences wound discharge and periprosthetic infection. *Clin Orthop Rel Res.*

30. Van de Belt H, Neut D, Schenk W, *et al.* (1999) ...Or not to treat? *Nature Medicine* 5:358–9.

31. Sanderson PJ. (1991) Infections in orthopaedic implants. *J Hosp Inf* 18(Suppl A):367–75.

32. LaPorte DM, Waldman BJ, Mont MA, Hungerford DS. (1999) Infections associated with dental procedures in total hip arthroplasty. *J Bone Joint Surg* 81B:56–9.

33. Busscher HJ, Geertsema-Doornbusch GI, Everaert EPJM, *et al.* (1996) Biofilm formation and silicone rubber surface modification in the development of a total artificial larynx. In: Algaba J (ed.), *Surgery and Prosthetic Voice Restoration after Subtotal Laryngectomy*, Elsevier Science, Amsterdam, pp. 47–52.

34. Van Loosdrecht MCM, Lyklema J, Norde W, Zehnder AJB. (1990) Influences of interfaces on microbial activity. *Microbiol Rev* 54:75–87.

35. Neu TR, Dijk F, Verkerke GJ, *et al.* (1992) Scanning electron microscopy study of biofilms on silicone voice prostheses. *Cells Materials* 3:261–9.

36. Isaklar ZU, Darouiche RO, Landon GC, Beck T. (1996) Efficacy of antibiotics alone for orthopaedic device related infections. *Clin Orthop* 332:184–9.

37. Schierholz JM, Beuth J. (2001) Implant infections: a haven for opportunistic bacteria. *J Hosp Inf* 49:87–93.

38. Sugarman B, Young EJ. (1989) Infections associated with prosthetic devices: magnitude of the problem. *Infect Dis Clin North Am* 3:187–99.

39. Elek SD, Conen PE. (1957) The virulence of *Staphylococcus pyogenes* for man. A study of the problems of wound infection. *Br J Exp Pathol* 38:5735–86.

40. Lam J, Chan R, Lam K, Costerton JW. (1980) Production of mucoid micro-colonies by *Pseudomonas aeroginosa* within infected lungs in cystic fibrosis. *Infect Immun* 28:546–56.

41. Nickel JC, Rureska I, Wright JB, Costerton JW. (1985) Tobramycin resistance of *Pseudomonas aeroginosa* growing as a biofilm on urinary catheter material. *Antimicrob Agents Chemother* 27:619–24.

42. Christensen GD, Baddour LM, Hasty DL, *et al.* (1989) In: Bisno AL, Waldvogel FA (eds.), *Infections Associated with Indwelling Medical Devices*, American Society of Microbiology, Washington DC, pp. 27–59.

43. Charnley J. (1972) Postoperative infection after total hip replacement with special reference to air contamination in the operating room. *Clin Orthop* 87:167–87.

44. Lidwell OM, Lowbury EJ, Whyte W, *et al.* (1982) Effect of ultraclean air in operating rooms on deep sepsis in the joint after total hip or knee replacement. A randomized study. *British Med J* **285**:10–14.
45. Fitzgerald RH Jr, Nasser S. (1995) Infection following total hip arthroplasty. In: Callagghan JJ, Dennis DA, Paprosky WG, Rosenberg AG. (eds.), *Orthopaedic Knowledge Update, Hip and Knee Reconstruction*, American Academy of Orthopaedic Surgeons, Rosemont, pp. 157–61.
46. Tang L, Eaton JW. (1995) Inflammatory responses to biomaterials. *Am J Clin Pathol* **103**:466–71.
47. Davenport K, Keeley FX. (2005) Evidence for the use of silver-alloy-coated urethral catheters. *J Hosp Infect* **4**:298–303.
48. Masse A, Bruno A, Bosetti M, *et al.* (2000) Prevention of pin track infection in external fixation with silver coated pins: clinical and microbiological results. *J Biomed Mater Res (Part B)* **53**:600–4.
49. Van der Borden AJ, Maathuis PG, Engels E, *et al.* (2007) Prevention of pin tract infection in external stainless steel fixation frames using electric current in a goat model. *Biomaterials* **28**(12):2122–6.
50. Mahieu HF, Saene HF, Rosingh HJ, Schutte HK. (1986) Candida vegetations on silicone voice prostheses. *Arch Otolaryngol Head Neck Surg* **112**:321–5.
51. Nickel JC, Costerton JW, Mclean RJ, Olson M. (1994) Bacterial biofilms: influence on the pathogenesis, diagnosis and treatment of urinary tract infections. *J Antimicrob Chemother Suppl A* **33**:31–41.
52. Mayer KH, Schoenbaum SC. (1982) Evaluation and management of prosthetic valve endocarditis. *Prog Cardiovasc Dis* **25**:43–54.
53. Bengtson S, Blomgren G, Knutson K, *et al.* (1987) Hematogenous infection after knee arthroplasty. *Acta Orthop Scand* **58**:529–34.
54. Fitzgerald RH Jr, Jones DR. (1985) Hip implant infection. Treatment with resection arthroplasty and late total hip arthroplasty. *Am J Med* **78**:225–8.
55. Hunter G, Dandy D. (1977) The natural history of the patient with an infected total hip replacement. *J Bone Joint Surg* **59B**:293–7.
56. Maniloff G, Greenwald R, Laskin R, Singer C. (1987) Delayed postbacteremic prosthetic joint infection. *Clin Orthop* **223**:194–7.
57. Costerton JW. (2005) Biofilm theory can guide the treatment of device-related orthopaedic infections. *Clin Orthop* **437**:7–11.
58. Philips WC, Kattapuram SV. (1983) Efficacy of preoperative hip aspiration performed in the radiology department. *Clin Orthop* **179**:141–6.
59. Donlan RM. (2005) New approaches for the characterization of prosthetic joint biofilms. *Clin Orthop* **437**:12–19.
60. Tunney MM, Patrick S, Curran MD, *et al.* (1999) Detection of prosthetic hip infection at revision arthroplasty by immunofluorescence microscopy and PCR amplification of the bacterial 16S rRNA gene. *J Clin Microbiol* **37**:3281–90.

61. Tunney MM, Patrick S, Gorman SP, *et al.* (1998) Improved detection of infection in hip replacements. *J Bone Joint Surg* 80B:568–72.
62. Nelson CL, McLaren AC, McLaren SG, *et al.* (2005) Is aseptic loosening truly aseptic? *Clin Orthop* 437:25–30.
63. Ahlberg A, Carlsson AS, Lindberg L. (1978) Hematogenous infection in total joint replacement. *Clin Orthop* 137:69–75.
64. Klein NE, Cox CV. (1994) Wound problems in total knee arthroplasty. In: Fu FH, Harner CD, Vince KG (eds.), *Knee Surgery*, Vol 2. Williams & Wilkins, Philadelphia, pp. 1539–52.
65. Wilson MG, Kelley K, Thornhill TS. (1990) Infection as a complication of total knee-replacement arthroplasty. Risk factors and treatment in sixty-seven cases. *J Bone Joint Surg* 72A:878–83.
66. Jerry GJ Jr, Rand JA. (1988) Old sepsis prior to total knee arthroplasty. *Clin Orthop* 236:135–40.
67. Schmalzried TP, Amstutz HC, Au MK, Dorey FJ. (1992) Etiology of deep sepsis in total hip arthroplasty. The significance of haematogenous and recurrent infections. *Clin Orthop* 280:200–7.
68. Okhuijsen SY, Dhert WJA, Faro LMC, *et al.* (1998) De totale heupprothese in Nederland. *Ned Tijdschr Geneeskund* 142:1434–8.
69. Eftekhar NS. (1993) Postoperative wound infection. In: *Total Hip Arthroplasty*, Vol. 2, Mosby, St. Louis, pp. 1457–1504.
70. Levi AD, Dickman CA, Sonntag VK. (1997) Management of postoperative infections after spinal instrumentation. *J Neurosurg* 86:975–80.
71. Schwab FJ, Nazarian DG, Mahmud F, Michelsen CB. (1995) Effects of spinal instrumentation on fusion of the lumbosacral spine. *Spine* 20:2023–8.
72. Jasty M, Maloney WJ, Bragdon CR, *et al.* (1990) Histomorphological studies of the long-term skeletal responses to well fixed cemented femoral components. *J Bone Joint Surg* 72A:1220–9.
73. Dougherty SH, Simmons RL. (1982) Infections in bionic man: the pathobiology of infections in prosthetic devices — Part I. *Current Problems in Surgery* 19:217–64.
74. Jackson JH, Cochrane CG. (1988) Leukocyte induced tissue injury. *Hematol Oncol Clin North Am* 2:317–34.
75. Rissing JP. (1990) Animal models of osteomyelitis. Knowledge, hypothesis and speculation. *Infect Dis Clin North Am* 4:377–90.
76. Tsukayama DT. (1999) Pathophysiology of posttraumatic osteomyelitis. *Clin Orthop* 360:22–9.
77. Ritter MA, French MLV, Eitzen HE. (1975) Bacterial contamination of the surgical knife. *Clin Orthop* 108:158–60.
78. Mackay DC, Harrison WJ, Bates JH, Dickenson D. (2000) Audit of deep wound infection following hip fracture surgery. *J R Coll Surg Edinb* 45:56–9.

79. Ellenhorn JD, Smith DD, Schwarz RE, *et al.* (2005) Paint-only is equivalent to scrub-and-paint in preoperative preparation of abdominal surgery sites. *J Am Coll Surg* **5**:737–41.

80. Seal LA, Paul-Cheadle D. (2004) A systems approach to preoperative surgical patient skin preparation. *Am J Infect Control* **2**:57–62.

81. Kjonniksen I, Andersen BM, Sondenaa VG, Segadal L. (2002) Preoperative hair removal — a systematic literature review. *AORN J* **75**:928–38.

82. Blomgren G, Hoborn J, Nyström B. (1990) Reduction of contamination at total hip replacement by special working clothes. *J Bone Joint Surg* **72B**:985–7.

83. Lipp A, Edwards P. (2002) Disposable surgical face masks for preventing surgical wound infection in clean surgery. *Cochrane Database Syst Rev* **1**:CD002929.

84. Santos AM, Lacerda RA, Graziano KU. (2005) Evidence of control and prevention of surgical site infection by shoe covers and private shoes: a systematic literature review. *Rev Lat Am Enfermagem* **1**:86–92.

85. Tanner J, Parkinson H. (2002) Double gloving to reduce surgical cross-infection. *Cochrane Database Syst Rev* (3):CD003087.

86. Davis N, Curry A, Gambhir AK, *et al.* (1999) Intraoperative bacterial contamination in operations for joint replacement. *J Bone Joint Surg* **81B**:886–9.

87. Fitzgerald RH Jr. (1992) Total hip arthroplasty sepsis. Prevention and diagnosis. *Orthop Clin North America* **23**:259–64.

88. Drabu YJ, Miller T. (1998) Importance of air quality and related factors in the prevention of infection in orthopaedic implant surgery. *J Hosp Infect* **39**:173–80.

89. Friberg BE, Friberg S, Burman LG. (1996) Zoned vertical ultraclean operating room ventilation. *Acta Orthop Scand* **67**:578–82.

90. Salvati EA, Robinson RP, Zeno SM, *et al.* (1982) Infection rates after 3175 total hip and total knee replacements performed with and without a horizontal unidirectional filtered air-flow system. *J Bone Joint Surg* **64A**:525–35.

91. Ritter MA, Eitzen HE, French MLV, Hartt JB. (1976) The effect that time, touch and environment have upon bacterial contamination of instruments during surgery. *Ann Surg* **184**:642–4.

92. Espehaug B, Engesaeter LB, Vollset SE, *et al.* (1997) Antibiotic prophylaxis in total hip arthroplasty. Review of 10,905 primary cemented total hip replacements reported to the Norwegian arthroplasty register, 1987 to 1995. *J Bone Joint Surg* **79B**:590–5.

93. Smyth ET, Humphreys H, Stacey A, *et al.* (2005) Survey of operating theatre ventilation facilities for minimally invasive surgery in Great Britain and Northern Ireland: current practice and considerations for the future. *J Hosp Inf* **2**:112–22.

94. Antti-Poika I, Josefsson G, Konttinen Y, *et al.* (1990) Hip arthroplasty infection. Current concepts. *Acta Orthop Scand* **61**:163–9.

95. Doyon F, Evrard J, Mazas F, Hill C. (1987) Long-term results of prophylactic cefazolin versus placebo in total hip replacement. *Lancet* **1**:860.

96. Hughes SPF, Want S, Darrell JH, *et al.* (1982) Prophylactic cefuroxime in total joint replacement. *Int Orthop* **6**:155–61.

97. Dent CD, Olson JW, Farish SE, *et al.* (1997) The influence of preoperative antibiotics on success of endosseous implants up to and including stage II surgery: a study of 2641 implants. *J Oral Maxillofac Surg* **55**:19–24.

98. Young RF, Lawner PM. (1987) Perioperative antibiotic prophylaxis for prevention of postoperative neurosurgical infections, A randomized clinical trial. *J Neurosurg* **66**:701–5.

99. Tang WM, Chiu KY, Ng TP, *et al.* (2003) Efficacy of a single dose of cefazolin as a prophylactic antibiotic in primary arthroplasty. *J Arthroplasty* **6**:714–8.

100. Wong ES. (1999) Surgical site infections. In: Mayhall CG (ed.), *Hospital Epidemiology and Infection Control,* Lippincott Williams & Wilkins, Philadelphia, pp. 189–210.

101. Duguid JP, Wallace AT. (1993) Air infection with dust liberated from clothing. *Lancet* **2**:845–9.

102. Thodis E, Passadakis P, Lyrantzopoouloos N, *et al.* (2005) Peritoneal catheters and related infections. *Int Urol Nephrol* **37**:379–93.

103. Walenkamp G. (2003) Surveillance of surgical-site infections in orthopedics. *Acta* **2**:172–4.

Case 1

Cardiopulmonary Bypass and Postoperative Organ Dysfunction

*Y. John Gu**

Cardiopulmonary bypass is one of the most popularly applied medical technologies of extracorporeal circulation for patients who need a heart operation. It is indicated to be employed during open-heart surgery to replace the function of the natural heart and lungs. The heart-lung machine is a machine system to be used for performing the cardiopulmonary bypass. It consists of a number of heart pumps, an oxygenator, and reservoirs and filters. Since the heart-lung machine contains a large surface area of nonphysiological synthetic materials, it induces tremendous blood activation and a whole-body inflammatory response that contributes to post-operative organ dysfunction. Research and development on optimizing the heart-lung machine system and cardiopulmonary bypass circuit will be of crucial importance in improving the care and post-operative organ function for cardiac surgical patients.

*Department of Biomedical Engineering, University Medical Center Groningen, A. Deusinglann 1, 9713 AV Groningen, The Netherlands.

Introduction

In heart surgery, for example, during coronary artery bypass graft-ing, the risk of inducing heart failure or cardiac infarction by the sur-gery itself may increase in high-risk patients. Moreover, functioning lungs may cover the operation area during open chest conditions, thus limiting the view and the handling of the surgeon. In these situ-ations the pump function of the heart and the function of the lungs can be taken over by a heart-lung machine. This chapter describes the so-called cardiopulmonary bypass, its advantages and disadvan-tages, its post-operative complications, and possibilities to prevent these complications.

The implementation of biomaterials in modern medicine has made possible the rapid progress of cardiothoracic surgery for at least the past five decades.[1] Among various achievements, the innovation and development of the heart-lung machine had enabled cardiac surgeons to make a cardiopulmonary bypass to replace the heart and lung function and to maintain the circulation during the so-called "open-heart" surgery.

Part I: Cardiopulmonary Bypass and Open-Heart Surgery

Under physiological circumstances, the heart functions as a pump driving blood through either the systemic circulatory system or the pulmonary circulatory system, whereas the lungs function largely for the oxygenation of blood within the pulmonary circulation.[2] During open-heart surgery a cardiopulmonary bypass using a heart-lung machine is usually necessary to replace the function of the heart and lungs.

The heart-lung machine consists of a main blood pump to replace the heart function and an oxygenator to replace the lung function during cardiopulmonary bypass (see Fig. 1). In addition, the heart-lung machine is equipped with a venous reservoir, a cardiotomy reser-voir, an integrated heat exchanger with the oxygenator, blood filters, venous and arterial cannulas, several monitoring apparatus, as well as other pumps to drive blood from the operation field to the heart-lung

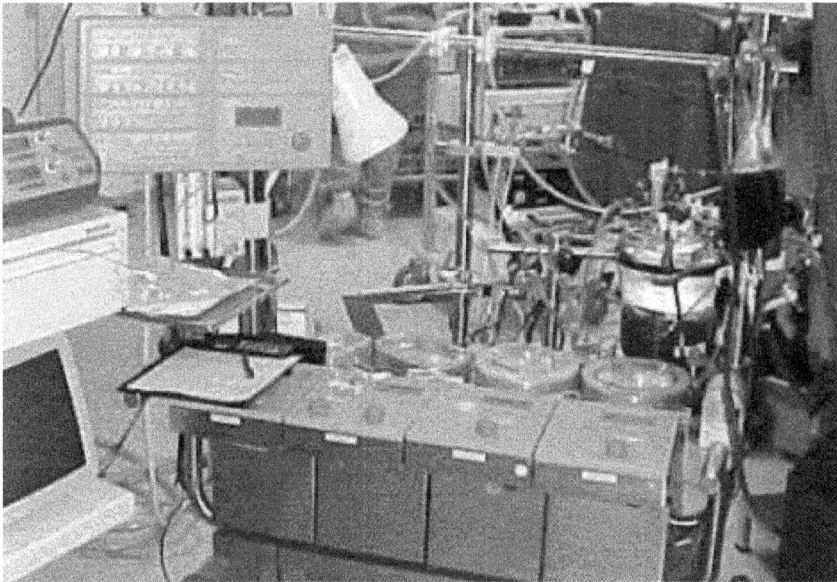

Fig. 1. The modern heart-lung machine and its related devices used for cardiopulmonary bypass during open-heart surgery.

machine, to decompensate the left ventricle through a vent, and to deliver cardioplegia to arrest the heart.[3,4]

Blood Pumps

The roller pump is the most popularly used blood pump in the heart-lung machine since the innovation of cardiopulmonary bypass. It drives blood by compressing plastic tubing between the roller and the backing plate as the roller turns in the raceway. The advantage of using roller pumps in the heart-lung machine is their predictable pump flow based on pump speed. However, the roller pump can over-pressurize the circuit and easily pump large quantities of air that are lethal to the patient. The centrifugal pump is a sort of the constrained vortex pump that drives blood by its centrifugal force. It does not over-pressurize the circuit because it is non-occlusive. Furthermore, it is less likely to pump a large amount of air to the patient.

The natural heart generates a strong pulse to the circulation, forming the so-called "pulsatile flow," with a measurable systolic and diastolic blood pressure in the aorta and the rest of the arterial system (see Fig. 2). However, the blood pumps commonly used in the heart-lung machine create a non-pulsatile flow, thus, only the mean arterial pressure is measurable during cardiopulmonary bypass when the natural heart is arrested. Theoretically, pulsatile flow has several advantages over non-pulsatile flow, including a better supply of hemodynamic energy to the microcirculation and improved organ perfusion and metabolism. Practically, it has not been widely applied because of the worry of adding increased complexity to the bypass circuit.

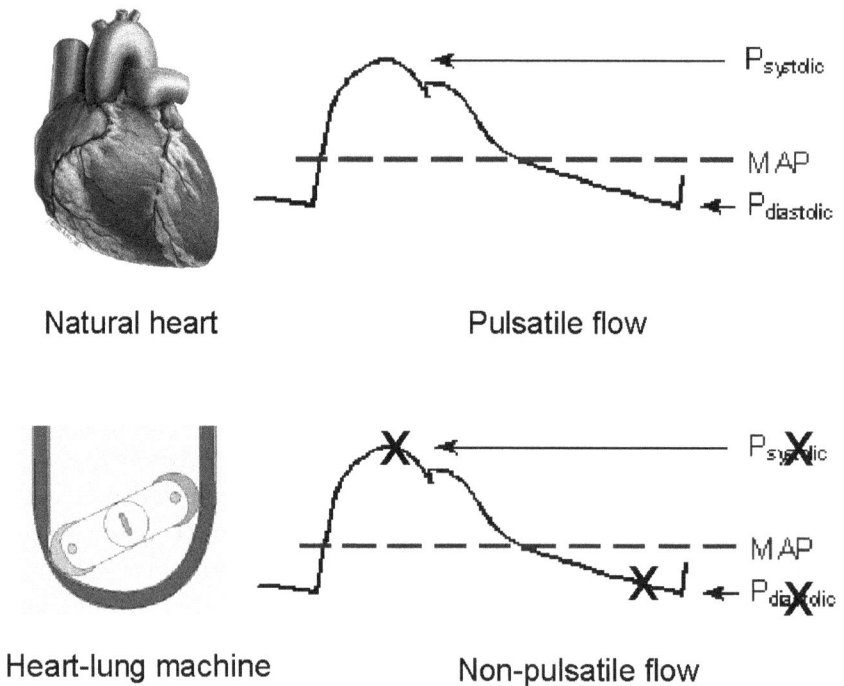

Fig. 2. Pulsatile versus non-pulsatile flow for cardiopulmonary bypass. Unlike the natural heart, the roller pump used in the heart-lung machine generates neither systolic nor diastolic pressure (P), but only the mean arterial pressure (MAP).

Oxygenators

Oxygenators are also called "artificial lungs." Basically, there are two types of oxygenators used in the heart-lung machine. The bubble oxygenator is the one made from a simple principle by which oxygen is just bubbled through the venous blood. After oxygenation, blood must be defoamed by an antifoam agent to remove foam and additional bubbles before the oxygenated blood is returned to the patient. Although the bubble oxygenator is efficient and inexpensive, and is indicated for patients with a short duration of cardiopulmonary bypass, it creates a direct blood-gas interface that will cause more blood damage, leading to post-operative organ dysfunction.

In contrast, the membrane oxygenator has been constructed to mimic the natural pulmonary anatomy by applying very thin membranes between blood and gas. The venous blood will be oxygenated through the principle of "permeability," thus having no direct blood contact with the gas (see Fig. 3). Membrane oxygenators can be divided further into the flat-sheet or hollow-fiber oxygenators based on their different constructions. The former is made of several synthetic membranes, usually silicone rubber sheets, organized in a cylindrical fashion, whereas the latter is made of microporous fibers, usually polypropylene, packed together in a parallel fashion. Nowadays, the hollow-fiber membrane oxygenator is the most commonly used oxygenator. However, due to the plasma leakage problem of the hollow fiber as a result of its pore structure, the flat-sheet membrane oxygenator is usually chosen when a longer duration of extracorporeal membrane oxygenation (ECMO) is indicated, such as in post-operative lung dysfunction (described later).

Part II: Postoperative Organ Dysfunction

Organ dysfunction, especially involving vital organs such as the heart, lung, brain, kidney, and the gastrointestinal system, is encountered relatively more frequently after open-heart surgery with cardiopulmonary bypass than with other types of surgery. This is due to the fact that along with the generalized surgical trauma caused by

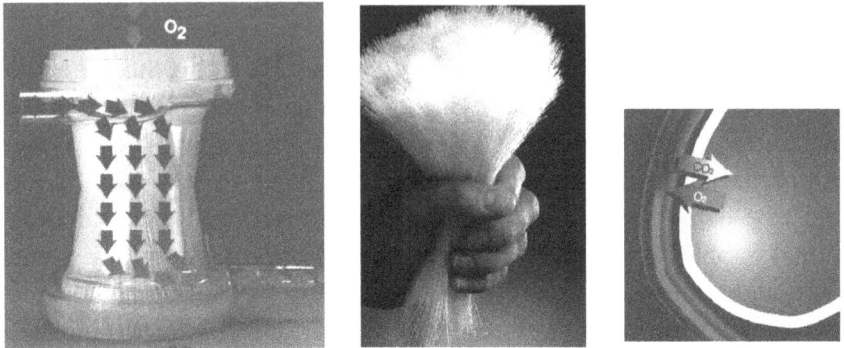

Fig. 3.   A membrane oxygenator made of hollow fibers (copyright Terumo Corporation).

any major operation, the use of cardiopulmonary bypass, with its large surface area of blood contact with non-physiological synthetic materials in the heart-lung machine, induces an additional inflammatory response, which may further contribute to post-operative organ dysfunction.

Heart

The myocardial ischemic/reperfusion injury associated with cardiopulmonary bypass, as well as the surgical insult to the heart and the underlying heart disease(s), can make the heart very sick during the early post-operative period. The most dangerous cardiac dysfunction after cardiopulmonary bypass is called the post-operative low cardiac output syndrome or postcardiotomy cardiogenic shock, which is characterized by reduced cardiac output, low blood pressure, poor left ventricular function, and compromised hemodynamics. This syndrome occurs in approximately 2% to 6% of patients who undergo open-heart surgery with cardiopulmonary bypass.[5] Usually, the low cardiac output syndrome is diagnosed if the patient cannot be weaned from cardiopulmonary bypass or experiences pump failure in the early post-operative period because of hemodynamic compromise. Furthermore, this syndrome is also diagnosed if the patient requires inotropic medication to maintain the systolic blood pressure above 90 mmHg and the cardiac output above 2.2 L/min/m^2 in the intensive care unit.

Mechanical circulatory support is an effective method to treat the postcardiotomy cardiogenic shock if the patient fails to respond to pharmacological inotropic support (see Fig. 4). The primary choice of mechanical circulatory support will be the intra-aortic balloon pump (IABP), which uses the principle of counterpulsation in the diastolic phase of each cardiac cycle. Benefits of this technique include augmentation of diastolic coronary perfusion pressure, reduction of systolic afterload, and an increase in cardiac output. Although IABP is an attractive form of circulatory support for a patient undergoing cardiac surgery, because of its ease of insertion and removal, this support system only yields a modest increase in cardiac output and does not displace a significant volume. Failure of the IABP to improve hemodynamic performance of the failing heart should prompt consideration of a rapid institution of a ventricular assist device (VAD). An ideal VAD should be able to be implanted and explanted easily and rapidly, permit uni- or biventricular assist, have minimal anticoagulation requirements, provide maximal unloading of the ventricle, be suitable to maintain an intermediate length of support up to a week, and be easy to convert to a long-term device. The pulsatile catheter (PUCA) pump developed at the University of Groningen is such a device that is to meet the above-mentioned criteria. Details about the PUCA pump, as well as other long-term mechanical circulatory support devices, will be described in the next chapter.

Lung

Lung injury or dysfunction after cardiopulmonary bypass is one of the most frequent complications after cardiac surgery.[6] It is caused by a combination of both bypass-associated factors such as blood-material interaction, hemodilution, hypothermia and ischemic/reperfusion, as well as non-bypass associated factors such as anesthesia

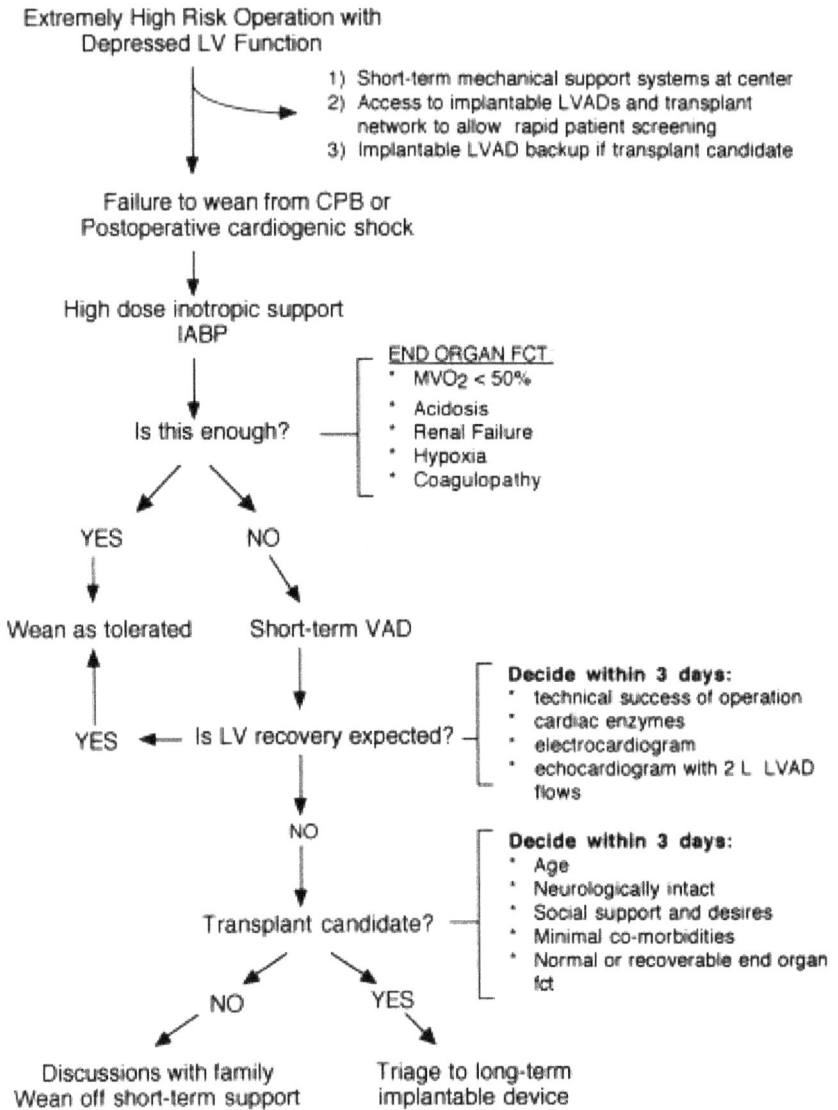

Fig. 4. Clinical algorithm for the management of postcardiotomy cardiogenic shock. (CPB = cardiopulmonary bypass; FCT, fct = function; IABP = intra-aortic balloon counterpulsation; LV = left ventricular; LVAD = left ventricular assist device; MVO_2 = myocardial oxygen consumption; VAD = ventricular assist device.) (Cited from reference 5 with permission from the publisher.)

and surgical trauma. Usually, post-operative lung dysfunction is reflected in a poor pulmonary gas exchange function, which can be diagnosed through numerous parameters, such as the alveolar-arterial oxygen pressure difference (P[A-a]O2), intrapulmonary shunt function, the degree of pulmonary edema and extravascular lung water, lung compliance, and pulmonary vascular resistance. Significantly increased P(A-a)O2 and pulmonary shunt fraction, together with decreased functional residual capacity and carbon monoxide transfer factor, have been observed in patients after cardiopulmonary bypass. Reduced lung gas exchange function after bypass is often the consequence of increased pulmonary capillary permeability, which is closely related to the formation of pulmonary edema, alveolar protein accumulation, and trans-pulmonary leukocyte sequestration. Under physiological circumstances, the lung capillaries are capable of holding a large amount of leukocytes, particularly the polymorphnuclear neutrophils (PMNs). These PMNs do not interact with the lung endothelium and only transit in the intravascular space forming a so-called "marginating" poor. During cardiopulmonary bypass, when blood flow passing through the lung is reduced (not stopped, because of the supply of the bronchial artery), there is an increased PMN-endothelium interaction, which will in turn result in the activation of both PMNs and endothelial cells and release of pro-inflammatory mediators, such as granular enzymes, oxygen free radicals, and cytokines. One of the most important enzymes released by PMNs is called elastase which is capable of degrading lung elastin and fibronectin, leading to lung injury.

Acute respiratory distress syndrome (ARDS) is one of the most severe forms of post-operative lung dysfunction with impaired oxygenation. This functional lung injury is identified histologically as diffuse damage to the alveolar-capillary unit. Disruption of the endothelial barrier in the pulmonary alveolocapillary membrane leads to noncardiogenic pulmonary edema through increased vascular permeability. Patients with post-operative ARDS are often treated with ECMO, which is a technique of adaptation of conventional cardiopulmonary bypass and mechanical circulatory support.

Brain

Post-operative cerebrovascular accidents, also called "stroke," occur in about 2% to 5% of patients after open-heart surgery.[7] Cardiopulmonary bypass may cause embolic cerebral infarction from air boluses, intracardiac clots, calcified debris, or foreign materials in the heart-lung machine circuit. Operations performed at normothermia have a higher incidence of stroke than those performed at moderate hypothermia. A lower perfusion pressure of less than 50 to 60 mmHg in the mean arterial pressure may also contribute. Furthermore, elderly patients or patients with carotid artery stenosis or an atheromatous macroemboli from the ascending aorta and aortic arch may be at high risk of a stroke during and after cardiopulmonary bypass.

In addition to stroke, a much larger population of patients suffer from neurocognitive dysfunction after heart surgery, which is likely associated with a generalized inflammatory response to cardiopulmonary bypass and increased permeability of the blood-brain barrier. The incidence of cognitive decline is believed to be around 50% to 80% at hospital discharge, 20% to 50% at six weeks and 10% to 30% at six months after operation.[7]

Kidney

Kidney dysfunction, or renal failure, after cardiac surgery has a significant influence on postoperative morbidity and mortality. Low cardiac output during and after cardiopulmonary bypass reduces renal perfusion pressure and causes angiotensin II production and renin release, which may further decrease renal blood flow. Kidneys, already compromised by pre-operative disease and the bypass-associated injury, are particularly sensitive to ischemic injury secondary to low cardiac output and hypotension. Post-operative renal dysfunction is usually treated with either hemofiltration or hemodialysis.[8] The former is aimed to remove the over-loaded fluid volume accumulated in the body as a result of cardiopulmonary bypass, whereas the latter is applied to help remove some specific metabolites or even toxic substances that are normally removed by the kidney. Technically, hemofiltration is a sort of ultrafiltration of blood plasma that is driven across a semi-permeable membrane by a pressure gradient, whereas hemodialysis works by circulating the blood through a special dialyzer or filter via osmotic differences between the blood and solute sides of the membrane. A combination of continuous venovenous hemofiltration and continuous venovenous hemodialysis is often used to treat severe acute renal dysfunction after cardiac surgery.

Gastrointestinal Organs

Since cardiopulmonary bypass also results in poor perfusion of the gastrointestinal organs, such as the stomach, gut, pancreas and liver, postoperative dysfunction associated with these organs may also occur, with an estimation of 0.5% to 3%. However, once it has occurred and developed into serious complications such as gastrointestinal bleeding, pancreatitis, cholecystitis, as well as mesenteric ischemia, the mortality rate can be as high as 20% to 80%. In patients with prolonged duration of cardiopulmonary bypass and prolonged aortic cross-clamping, gastrointestinal complications are more likely to occur. Although splanchnic organ function and hepatocellular integrity are likely affected by a prolonged period of perfusion, liver failure is rarely encountered after cardiopulmonary bypass unless the patient develops multiple organ failure.

Bleeding

Bleeding, or the tendency to bleed, is still one of the most frequent complications encountered after cardiopulmonary bypass surgery. Contact of blood with the foreign biomaterials in the heart-lung machine, as well as the non-physiological flow pattern and shear stresses created by the heart-lung machine, may cause platelet dysfunction and consumption of various components of coagulation and fibrinolytic cascades. These are believed to be the main causes of post-operative bleeding. Moreover, the systemic heparinization to facilitate the use of the heart-lung machine may further predispose patients with post-operative bleeding diathesis. Furthermore, the current successful antiplatelet and/or antithrombin therapies for patients with coronary artery diseases add additional risk of bleeding once these patients need to be operated on with cardiopulmonary bypass.

Whole-Body Inflammatory Response

Whole-body inflammatory response to cardiopulmonary bypass, which is different from a local inflammation, is a unique form of inflammatory response to both surgical trauma and the use of the heart-lung machine (see Fig. 5).[9] This generalized inflammatory response is characterized by a systemic activation of cellular and humoral cascades, including stimulation of complement and

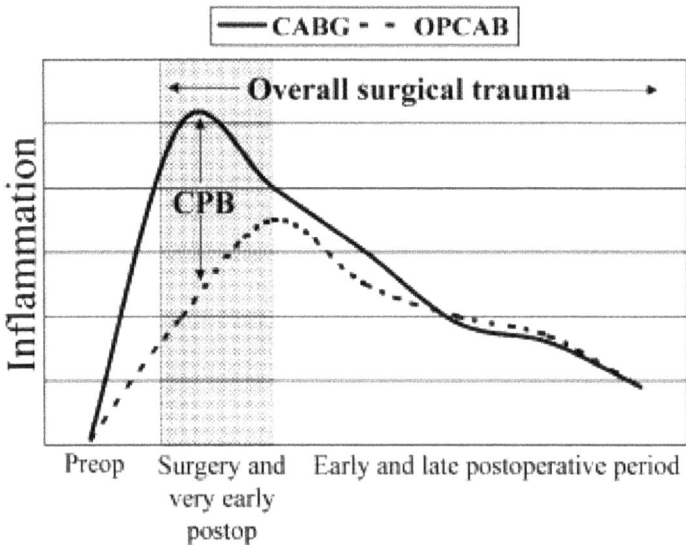

Fig. 5. Postoperative inflammation caused by both the cardiopulmonary bypass (CPB) and overall surgical trauma. Note the difference between the coronary artery bypass grafting (CABG) surgery and the off-pump coronary artery bypass (OPCAB) surgery, by which the latter is operated without CPB. (Cited from reference 9 with permission from the publisher.)

coagulation systems, activation of leukocytes and platelets, and inter-action between leukocytes and endothelial cells, as well as increased production of inflammatory mediator and cytokines. Clinically, patients are manifesting with post-operative fever, increased circulating leuko-cyte count and a general capillary leak syndrome. Post-operatively, this systemic inflammatory response syndrome can be well tolerated in a vast majority of low-risk patients. In high-risk patients, how-ever, this syndrome may contribute to several adverse post-operative outcomes, such as renal, pulmonary and neurological complications, as discussed previously. Multiple organ failure may also occur as an extreme consequence of whole-body inflammatory response.

Summary

Nowadays, with advanced catheter technology and rapid progress in interventional cardiology, patients referred to cardiac surgery with cardiopulmonary bypass are usually older and sicker, having poorer pre-operative heart function or more extensive disease than in earlier decades. Thus, a more physiological cardiopulmonary bypass circuit, with improved biomaterials and golden standard blood compatibility, will play a crucial role in reducing post-operative organ dysfunction, especially in high-risk patients.

References

1. Edmunds LH. (2004) Cardiopulmonary bypass after 50 years. *Editorial, N Engl J Med* 351:1603–6.
2. Martini FH. (2006) *Fundamentals of Anatomy and Physiology*. Pearson Educa-tion, Inc., publishing as Pearson Benjamin Cummings, 7th ed.
3. Kay PH, Munsch CM. (2004) *Techniques in Extracorporeal Circulation*, 4th ed. Arnold, London.
4. Turina M. (2006) *Multimedia Manual of Cardiothoracic Surgery* (MMCTS), The European Association for Cardio-thoracic Surgery, http://mmcts.ctsnet journals.org.
5. DeRose JJ Jr, Umana JP, Argenziano M, *et al.* (1997) Improved results for post-cardiotomy cardiogenic shock with the use of implantable left ventricular assist devices. *Ann Thorac Surg* 64:1757–62.

6. Taggart DP, el-Fiky M, Carter R, *et al.* (1993) Respiratory dysfunction after uncomplicated cardiopulmonary bypass. *Ann Thorac Surg* **56**:1123–8.
7. Newman MF, Kirchner JL, Phillips-Bute B, *et al.* (2001) Longitudinal assessment of neurocognitive function after coronary artery bypass surgery. *N Engl J Med* **344**:395–402.
8. Joy MS, Matzke GR, Frye RF, Palevsky PM. (1998) Determinants of vancomycin clearance by continuous venovenous hemofiltration and continuous venovenous hemodialysis. *Am J Kidney Dis* **31**:1019–27.
9. Biglioli P, Cannata A, Alamanni F, *et al.* (2003) Biological effects of off-pump vs. on-pump coronary artery surgery: focus on inflammation, hemostasis and oxidative stress. *Eur J Cardiothorac Surg* **24**:260–9.

Case 2

Mechanical Circulatory Support Systems

G. Rakhorst* and M.E. Erasmus[†]

Heart failure can be defined as a situation in which the pump function of the heart is not able to maintain the proper functioning of the vital organs, or in other words, the heart cannot generate enough blood pressure and flow to guarantee adequate organ perfusion. In case pharmaceutical and interventional cardiologic therapies like medication, intracoronary balloon dilatation or stent placement fail in treatment of severe heart failure, mechanical circulatory support of the diseased heart may become a life-saving therapy. In order to understand heart failure and mechanical circulatory support, the reader must be aware of the natural anatomy of the heart and its functioning and the different types of blood pumps that can be applied to assist a failing heart.

*Department of BioMedical Engineering, University Medical Center Groningen, A. Deusinglaan 1, 9713 AV Groningen, The Netherlands.
[†]Thorax Department, University Medical Center Groningen, Hanzeplein 1, 9713 GZ Groningen, The Netherlands.

Introduction

The heart contains four chambers (see Fig. 1), the left atrium (LA), the left ventricle (LV), the right atrium (RA) and the right ventricle (RV). The LA collects oxygen-enriched blood from the lung veins and transports this to the LV, from which it will be ejected into the systemic circulation (aorta). The RA collects oxygen-poor blood from the caval veins and transports this to the RV, which ejects this into the pulmonary circulation (pulmonary artery). Heart valves between the atria and the ventricles (atrio-ventricular (A-V) valves: right side tricuspid valves, left side bicuspid valves), and between the

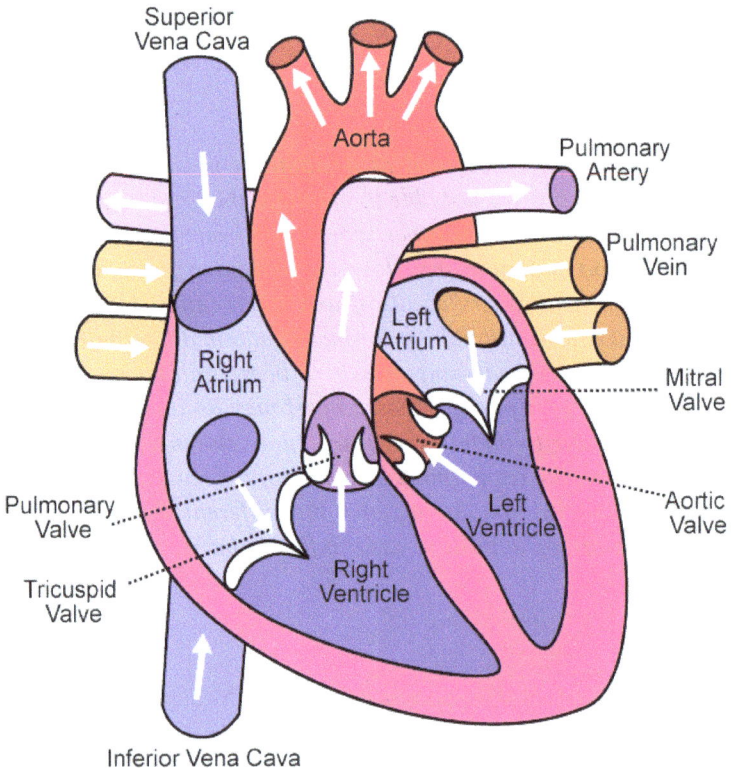

Fig. 1. Schematic drawing of the heart (from Wikipedia).

LV and aorta and RV and pulmonary artery (semi-lunar valves: left side aortic valves, right side pulmonary artery valves) guide the blood in a unidirectional way (see Fig. 1). The A-V valves differ in size and shape from the semi-lunar valves, as well as from each other. Their leaflets are connected with numerous small tendons (chordae tendinea) to the papillary muscles of the ventricular wall. The aortic and pulmonary artery valves are quite similar.

The heart muscle itself receives oxygen enriched blood from the aorta, through the right and left coronary arteries. The orifices of these vessels are located just behind (distal) the aortic valve in the proximal part of the aorta (aorta ascendens). The left coronary artery divides into two branches, the left anterior descending coronary artery (LAD) and the left circumflex coronary artery (LCX). The collaterals of right coronary artery meet with the LCX in the base of the heart and its main branch, the right posterior descending coronary artery (RPD) meets with capillaries of the LAD in the apical region of the heart (see Fig. 2).

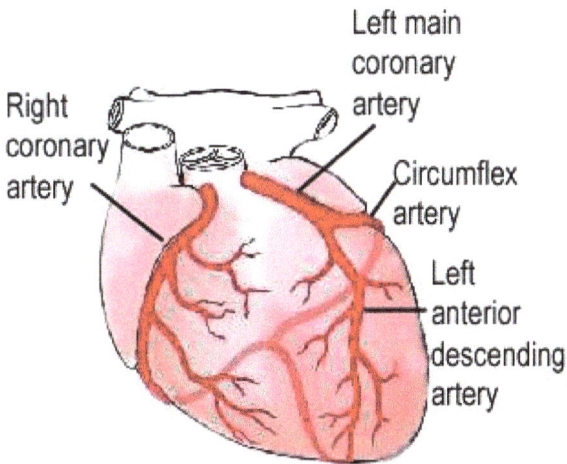

Fig. 2. Schematic drawing of the heart showing the coronary artery system (From: http://www.clevelandclinic.org/heartcenter/images/guide/disease/cad/coronary%20 arteries.jpg).

The left ventricular wall (myocardium) is thicker than the right ventricular wall and generates five times more pressure (125 mm Hg versus 25 mm Hg, respectively).

In case the blood flow in the coronary artery system is hampered, for example by a atherosclerotic plaque or a blood clot, the tissue distal from the stenosis will receive less blood and becomes short of oxygen (ischemic). If this situation continues, this tissue might die (cardiac infarction) due to a lack of oxygen, resulting in a part of the non-functional myocardium: the infarcted area does not contract and the cells of the conductive tissue of the heart might become non-functional as well, resulting in irregular heart beats. As a consequence, the pump function of the heart will diminish, resulting in decreased stroke volume (volume of blood that is ejected during every contraction) and decreased cardiac output (CO = stroke volume × heart frequency/minute). In a case where the situation has established itself very quickly it is called acute ischemic heart failure. In a case where it developed gradually it is called chronic ischemic heart failure. In chronic ischemic heart failure the left ventricle will dilate gradually, causing the vicious circle of increased wall stress (and oxygen consumption) and annulus dilation of the mitral valve, causing regurgitation.

Primary valvular diseases can also induce heart failure. In a case where the aortic valve becomes stenotic by calcification, the LV has to generate a higher pressure to eject the same amount of blood through the rigid semi-lunar valve. The LV myocardium will increase in thickness to generate the required pressure, resulting in a situation called pressure overload. If the aortic valve leaks there will be a volume overload, causing the heart to dilate. Acute aortic insufficiency can be lethal; chronic insufficiency leads to heart failure. Finally, if the mitral valve leaflets do not close properly, blood will be partly ejected backwards to the atria instead of forward to the aorta, resulting in similar heart failure conditions. As a consequence, the heart will increase its frequency in order to compensate for the loss of blood through the leaking heart valve. When the leakage is too much the right ventricle will decompensate.

General Therapies for Heart Failure

I. Acute and Chronic Ischemic Heart Failure

Medication:

- decreasing workload by decreasing blood pressure (ACE inhibitors) and diuretics
- prevention of blood clot formation with anticoagulants
- reduction of oxygen demand by decreasing heart rate with β-blockers.

Operation

- biventricular pacing in some cases
- in case of acute coronary syndrome, lysis of clots with enzymes or coronary stent
- in case of chronic ischemic heart failure, coronary stent placement or coronary artery bypass surgery with or without mitral valve surgery
- heart remodeling operation combined with mitral valve surgery
- end-stage heart failure: mechanical circulatory support.

II. Valvular Diseases (Aortic Stenosis/Insufficiency or Mitral Insufficiency)

Operation

- replacement of the stenotic or insufficient heart valve by a valve prosthesis
- enhancement of valve closure of the A-V valves by surgical valve or annulus reconstruction techniques
- end-stage heart failure: mechanical circulatory support.

Mechanical Circulatory Support

Mechanical circulatory support systems (MCSSs), ventricular assist devices (VADs) or heart assist devices are blood pumps that support or replace the pump function of the heart. When connected to the circulatory system these pumps influence the workload of the diseased heart either by: direct unloading (decreasing the wall stress by pumping blood out of the heart into the circulatory system); increasing the oxygen delivery to the heart (increasing the coronary flow); or by a realizing a combination of these two methods. Depending on the clinical situation (acute versus chronic heart failure), the intended use (short-term versus long-term assist) and the costs involved, various devices meet the medical and technical needs.

MCSSs can be categorized in various ways:

A – Total artificial heart and ventricular assist devices
1. Total Artificial Heart (TAH). The idea of developing a total artificial heart (TAH) originates from the early 1950s, when heart transplantation suffered from immune responses and acute rejection and it was assumed that artificial hearts could overcome this problem. A TAH is an implantable blood pump that replaces the natural ventricles. The TAH is composed of two blood pumps, a left and a right blood chamber, which aspire blood from the left and right atria and eject it into the aorta and pulmonary artery. The blood chamber is compressed electromechanically or pneumatically and heart valve prostheses, which replace the natural valves, guide the blood in a uni-directional flow. In 1971 Kwann-Gett[1] performed animal experiments with a TAH that consisted of two hemispherical membrane pumps (see Fig. 3, left). In the 1980s that heart became known as the Jarvik-7, produced by a company called Symbion. This TAH was activated by a pneumatic heart driver that could operate in an ECG-triggered mode (P-wave triggered) and in a set pump frequency. Later this pump was produced by CardioWest, a spin-off company of the University of Utah, and today it is marketed as the SynCardia TAH (see Fig. 3, right). Anticoagulation plays a pivotal rule in the functioning of a TAH. Improper anticoagulation leads to thrombus formation, resulting in stroke and (multi)organ failure. The transcutaneous pneumatic drive lines inhibit the risk of infection.

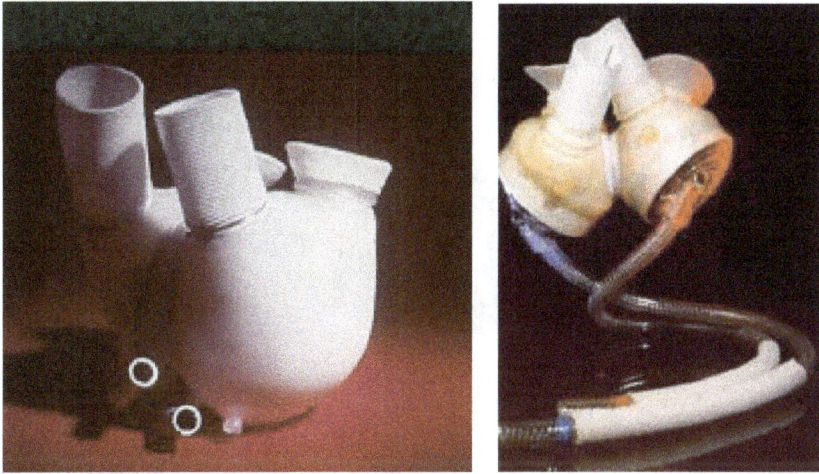

Fig. 3.   Picture of the Kwan-Gett TAH (left) and the SynCardia TAH (right).

The advantage of a pneumatically driven TAH is the fact that air is compressible. When a pneumatic TAH is faced with an increased venous return, the membrane that divides the blood pump into an air chamber and a blood chamber is pushed deeper into the air chamber, thus increasing the volume of the blood chamber. As a consequence, the next pump ejection delivers a higher stroke volume to the circulation, following the reaction upon increased venous inflow of the natural heart, which is described as the Frank–Starling Law.

To overcome the problem of infection caused by the pneumatic drive lines, various pump TAH designs followed that used a built in electromotor and pusher plates that activate emptying and filling of the blood chambers. The electromotor receives its energy either by transcutaneous drive lines or by implantable rechargable batteries and induction coils. The AbioCor TAH produced by Abiomed is electrohydraulically activated (see Fig. 4).

2. Ventricular Assist Devices (VADs). A new way of assisting heart failure was established when TAH technology was applied in such a way that the failing heart could be kept in place. VADs represent

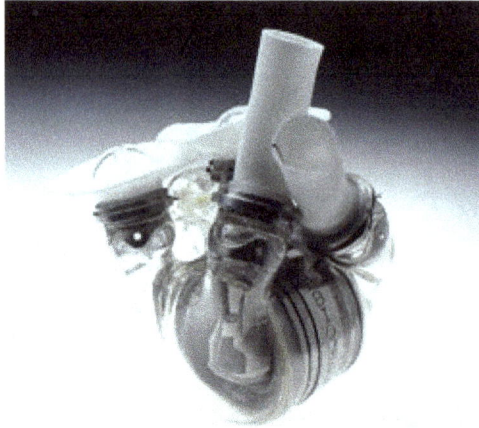

Fig. 4.   Picture of the AbioCor (with permission of Abiomed).

a number of blood pumps that are connected to the main blood vessels using in and outflow cannulas. VADs can be totally implanted (Novacor, HeartMate) or placed on the outside of the body (paracorporeally, Berlin Heart, MEDOS, etc.). VADs can be categorized into Left Ventricular Assist Devices (LVADs), Right Ventricular Assist Devices (RVADs), or Bi-Ventricular Assist Devices (BiVADs).

B – Pulsatile versus non-pulsatile blood pumps
The TAH and VADs described so far belong to the so-called membrane pumps. Membrane pumps generate a pulsatile flow. Like in the natural heart, pump ejection takes place when the pump pressure is high enough to open the outflow valve. After the blood chamber has been emptied, the blood chamber will be enlarged by moving the membrane, thus closing the outflow valve and opening the inflow valve.

Centrifugal pumps (see Fig. 5) generate a continuous flow. By rotating a number of impeller blades inside a blood chamber, blood is centrifuged from the center of the blood chamber towards the outside of the pump. Centrifugal pumps do not require heart valves and are easier and cheaper to manufacture. Although rotary blood pumps

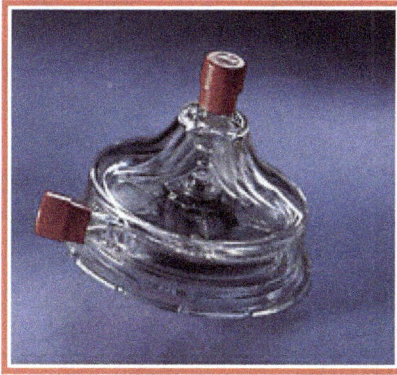

Fig. 5.   The Bio Pump (manufactured by Medtronics).

can be made implantable, most types are placed in extracorporeal circuits like heart-lung machines and Extra Corporeal Membrane Oxygenation machines (ECMO) as an alternative to roller pumps.

C – Closed-chest versus open-chest pump applications

Most VADs need major surgery for positioning. The chest has to be opened (thoracotomy) to connect the in- and outflow cannulas to the heart and main blood vessels. Transcutaneous blood pumps can be positioned under closed-chest conditions. Most of them can be introduced into the ventricular cavity through a peripheral superficial artery, such as the axillary, subclavian or femoral artery. These catheter-type blood pumps are meant to assist the heart under emergency conditions in order to stabilize the hemodynamics of a heart failure patient. The following pumps belong to these so-called transarterial blood pumps:

1. *Intra Aortic Balloon Pump (IABP)*

The IABP (see Fig. 6) consists of a large balloon (40–80 ml) placed on top of a catheter. The balloon catheter is inserted through the femoral artery and placed in the proximal part of the aorta. During the contraction of the heart (systole), when the blood is ejected from the LV into the aorta, the balloon is deflated by the vacuum generated by the

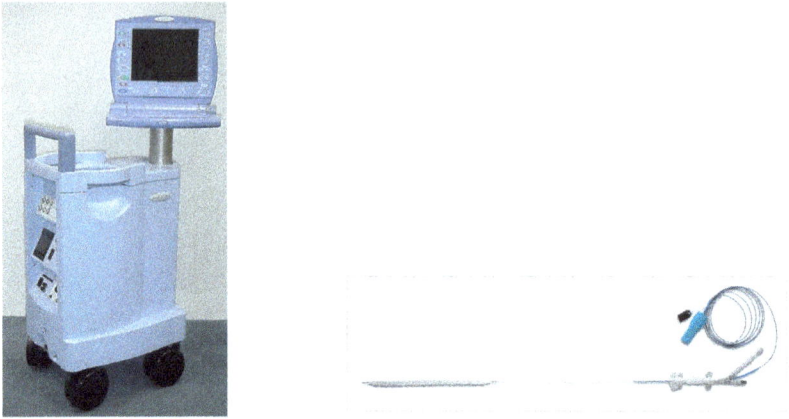

Fig. 6. Picture of the Arrow A-cath IABP driving console (left) and IABP catheter (right), with permission of Arrow International, USA.

IABP driver. When the heart is filled with blood (diastole) the balloon is filled with helium, thus generating a blood stream towards the heart (counter pulsation) that equals the replaced blood volume of the balloon. The IABP balloon reduces the afterload of the heart when the balloon is deflated by creating a space that has to be filled with blood when the balloon is emptied. The IABP needs ECG triggering. When the balloon is inflated during systole, the coronary arteries are compressed and the heart has to eject its blood against an obstruction caused by the inflated balloon, resulting in a higher workload, instead of unloading the failing heart. The effect of the IABP on the coronary artery flow is optimal when balloon inflation takes place during diastole, when the coronary arteries are open. Although the IABP is called a pump, it does not remove blood from the ventricles into the main blood vessels. The IABP is used 200,000 times per year worldwide, and is therefore the most used left ventricular assist device.

2. *PulseCath*®

The PulseCath® (see Fig. 7) is composed of a 21 Fr (7 mm outer diameter) thin-walled catheter that is connected to a transparent

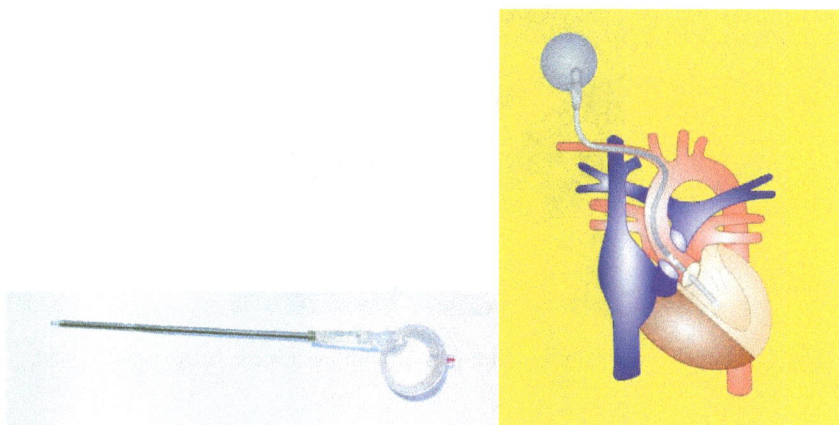

Fig. 7. Picture of the PulseCath® (left) and schematic drawing of the positioning of the PulseCath® during operation (right, with permission of Intra-Vasc BV, the Netherlands).

rigid single-port membrane pump. The pump is positioned through the subclavian artery, or during open chest conditions through the aortic wall, with its tip placed into the left ventricular cavity, thus positioning the aortic valve around the catheter tip. Approximately 6 cm from the tip, a combined in- and outflow valve guides the blood from the LV towards the membrane pump, and from the membrane pump through the same catheter towards the aorta. The PulseCath® produced by Intra-Vasc, a spin-off company of the University of Groningen, the Netherlands, can be activated by regular, commercially available IABP or other pneumatic heart drivers. The 21 Fr PulseCath® can generate a pump flow of 2.5–3 L/min.[2] When the pump operates in an ECG-triggered way, it combines direct ventricular unloading with counter pulsation. In case of irregular heart frequencies the pump can be operated on a set pump frequency.

3. Impella Miniaxial Blood Pumps

The Impella miniaxial blood pumps (see Fig. 8) consist of a high-speed rotor pump (25,000 rpm), which is electromagnetically activated,

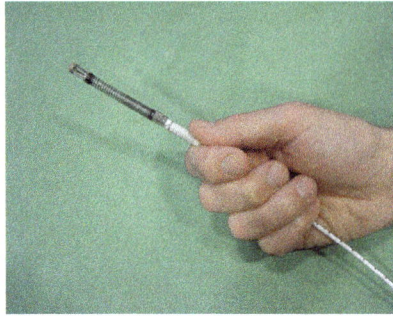

Fig. 8. Impella miniaxial catheter pump (with permission of Abiomed, USA).

placed on top of a catheter. Like the PulseCath, the Impella miniaxial pump is positioned through the aortic wall, the subclavian artery or femoral artery, with its tip in the left ventricular cavity.[3] Blood is sucked from the LV and ejected into the aorta in a continuous way, thus directly unloading the LV myocardium. The Impella RV support system sucks blood out of the RV and ejects it into the pulmonary artery (PA). Besides a 21 Fr version, Impella has a 12 Fr version that can be used for cardiac interventions like high-risk PTCA procedures.

4. *Tandem Heart*

The Tandem Heart is a catheter pump system that can be connected between the femoral vein and femoral artery.[4] The tip of the venous catheter is positioned in the right atrium and punctured through the interatrial septum into the LA. An external centrifugal pump sucks blood out of the LA and ejects it into the femoral artery.

D – Pump application

Blood pumps can also be categorized according to their application:

1) Bridge to the OR room. Pump systems that belong to this category are meant to stabilize the hemodynamic condition of acute ischemic heart failure patients. The pumps used are meant for short-term support (from a few hours to 3–5 days) and allow fast positioning. Most of these pumps belong to the trans-arterial

blood pumps, described earlier in this chapter, such as IABP, Impella and PulseCath.

2) Bridge to recovery. More or less by accident it was noticed that some patients who were treated with a Berlin Heart to bridge the time needed to find a suitable donor heart, were in rather good condition at the time of the scheduled surgery. Hetzer *et al.* described this phenomenon as recovery.[5] Patients suffering from viral myocarditis also recovered from their illness with the help of mechanical cardiac support. The Helmholtz Institute in Aachen, Germany, developed a prototype of a so-called Ventricular Recovery Support System, the VERSUS: a totally implantable electromechanical blood pump with a stroke volume of 35 ml that generates a pump flow of 2.5–3.5 L/min (see Fig. 7, reference 6).

3) Bridge to heart transplantation. The first pump used to bridge a patient to heart transplantation (HTx) was the Jarvik-7. Although many universities all over the world are developing various types of TAHs, only the SynCardia TAH and the Abiomed can be clinically applied. The Pen-state BiVAD and HeartMate-EM LVADs are positioned in parallel with the heart between the LV and Ao and meant for long-term support. Because the native heart is kept in place, these pumps belong to the LVAD and BiVAD categories. The longest support with the Novacor is 5 years.[7]

4) Destination therapy. Heart transplantation has become a victim of its own success. Due to the growing possibilities to treat end-stage heart failure with replacement of the diseased heart with the heart of a donor, the demand for donor hearts by far exceeds the availability. Moreover, by the growing life expectancy of our population and the success of medical treatments, the age of patients that need HTx or MCSS is increasing as well. The Abiomed TAH is meant to support heart failure patients that do not meet the requirements of HTx and that can establish a good quality of life when their heart is replaced by a totally implantable blood pump. The Abiocor (see Fig. 4) is an electrohydraulically driven blood pump that consists of two hemispherical blood chambers. The pump medium is driven by a small rotor pump

from one chamber to the other, thus generating an alternating pump ejection. The pump has been applied clinically in 15 patients.[8]

E – Pump activation

As previously mentioned, blood pumps can be activated in different ways — pneumatically, electromechanically or electrohydraulically — requiring bulky external driving consoles or portable driving units and integrated energy transmission systems.

1) Pneumatic pumps. Pneumatic pumps either use air or helium to expand the air chamber of a membrane pump or to inflate a balloon catheter. The main advantage of air or gas is that it is compressible. Gas can pass through small tubes quickly, which makes pneumatic drivers suitable for following the ECG as a triggering signal. Due to the inertia of fluid, electrohydraulic pumps can only follow ECG triggering at low frequencies. Clinically applicable pneumatic driving consoles (IABP driver, MEDOS Heart Driver, etc.) consist of a compressor and a vacuum pump and a back-up system. Therefore, these systems are quite heavy and bulky and meant for long-term use. Portable systems have been developed that allow patients to move freely. These systems, however, can be applied for a few hours only.

2) Electrohydraulic pumps. Electrohydraulic pumps use mineral oil or water to move the membrane of a displacement pump (see Abiocor).

3) Electromagnetic pumps. Dr. Peer Portner designed a membrane pump in which the blood bag is compressed by two sets of springs that are attracted and rejected from each other by electromagnets.[9] The Novacor is too large to be implanted inside the chest. The pump is therefore placed in a pocket in the abdomen, near the diaphragm.

4) Electromechanical pumps. Electromechanical pumps move a spindle connected to a pusher plate using an electromotor. This type of pump motor is suitable to activate TAHs or LVADs. In the case of a TAH, both ventricles will be activated in an alternating way.

Conclusion

This chapter is meant to give the reader an impression of the developments in MCSS. More information can be gathered from numerous textbooks, as well as from the Internet. The role of rotary blood pumps is described rather briefly. Rotary blood pumps and miniaxial pumps are being developed by many research centers and are increasingly being clinically applied. More information on rotary blood pumps can be obtained from the website of the International Society for Rotary Blood Pumps and in various issues of *Artificial Organs*.[10]

References

1. Kwan-Gett CS, Van Kampen KR, Kawai J, *et al.* (1971) Results of total artificial heart implantation in calves. *J Thorac Cardiovasc Surg* **62**(6):880–9.
2. Mihaylov D, Rakhorst G, Van der Plaats A, *et al.* (2000) *In vivo* and *in vitro* experience with the PUCA-II, a single valved pulsatile catheter-pump. *Int J Artif Organs* **23**(10):697–702.
3. Meyns B, Stolinski J, Leunens V, *et al.* (2003) Left ventricular support by catheter-mounted axial flow pump reduces infarct size. *J Am Coll Cardiol* **41**(7):1087–95.
4. Vranckx P, Foley DP, De Feijter PJ, *et al.* (2003) Clinical introduction of the Tandemheart, a percutaneous left ventricular assist device, for circulatory support during high-risk percutaneous coronary intervention. *Int J Cardiovasc Intervent* **5**(1):35–9.
5. Hetzer R, Muller JH, Weng YG, *et al.* (2000) Midterm follow-up of patients who underwent removal of a left ventricular assist device after cardiac recovery from end-stage dilated cardiomyopathy. *J Thorac Cardiovasc Surg* **120**(5):843–53.
6. Jassawalla JS, Daniel MA, Chen H, *et al.* (1988) *In vitro* and *in vivo* testing of a totally implantable left ventricular assist system. *ASAIO-Trans* **34**(3):470–5.
7. Potapov EV, Weng Y, Drews T, *et al.* (2005) Longest time of support by the Novacor left ventricular assist device without pump exchange. *Ann Thorac Surg* **80**(6):2421.
8. Frazier OH, Dowling RD, Gray LA Jr, *et al.* (2004) The total artificial heart: where we stand. *Cardiology* **101**(1–3):117–21.
9. Tanaka A, Yoshizawa M, Abe K, *et al.* (2003) *In vivo* test of pressure head and flow rate estimation in a continuous-flow artificial heart. *Artif Organs* **27**(1):99–103.
10. Golding LAR (ed.). (2005) Heart failure and rotary blood pump summit. *Artificial Organs* **29**(7):517–91.

11. Martini FH (ed.). (2005) *Fundamentals of Anatomy and Physiology*. Prentice Hall, Englewood Cliffs, New Jersey, USA.
12. Merhige ME, Smalling RW, Cassidy D, *et al.* (1989) Effect of the hemopump left ventricular assist device on regional myocardial perfusion and function. Reduction of ischemia during coronary occlusion. *Circulation* 80(5 Pt 2):III158–66.

Biomaterial-related Infections in Orthopedic Implants

D. Neut* and R.L. Diercks[†]

Total joint arthroplasty is one of the most cost-effective surgical interventions of the last 50 years. With the development of new metallurgic, physical and chemical techniques, degenerated and destroyed joints, especially the hip and the knee, can be replaced by artificial joints. Patients are again capable to live a pain-free life, with a range of motion adequate for daily activities. On average, modern endoprostheses function in more than 90% of patients for 15 years without wear or loosening problems.

Aseptic loosening, as a result of wear and bone resorption, and infection, form the limits of a successful arthroplasty. New developments in osseo-integration, to promote incorporation of the prosthesis in the bone, and in passive (antibiotic) or active (immunologic) defense against microbial infection are the subject of intensive research. The latest developments are discussed in this chapter.

*Department of BioMedical Engineering, University Medical Center Groningen, A. Deusinglaan 1, 9713 AV Groningen, The Netherlands.
[†]Department of Orthopedics, University Medical Center Groningen, Hanzeplein 1, 9713 GZ Groningen, The Netherlands.

The Development of Total Hip Prostheses

Due to the crippling nature of degenerative arthritis, surgeons have been trying for well over a century to successfully treat this debilitating disease. There was an extensive search for material that could be utilized to resurface or even replace the hip. Several proposals and trials were made, including the use of muscles, fat, chromatized pig bladder, gold, magnesium and zinc. All met with failure. Surgeons and scientists were unable to find a material which was biocompatible with the body, and yet strong enough to withstand the tremendous forces placed on the hip joint.

In 1923, the first mold prosthesis was used for interpositional arthroplasty by the Norwegian-born American surgeon Marius Smith-Petersen[1,2] from Boston, Massachusetts. This glass mould interposition was intended to provide bone-implant movement on both the acetabular and femoral side of the implant. Unfortunately, glass, while proving biocompatible — and later also celluloid, Bakelite plastic, stainless steel and Pyrex — proved to be too brittle for the normal forces across the hip joint.[3] In 1938, Smith-Petersen implanted the first Vitallium mold, after its recent introduction to the dentistry market. This device provided the first predictable result in interpositional hip arthroplasty.

A dramatic improvement was made in 1936 when scientists manufactured a cobalt-chromium alloy which was almost immediately applied to orthopedics. This new alloy was both very strong and resistant to corrosion. While this new metal proved to be a great success, the actual resurfacing technique was found to be less than adequate. Frederick R. Thompson[4] (see Fig. 1) of New York, and Austin T. Moore[5] (see Fig. 2) of South Carolina, separately developed replacements for the entire ball of the hip.

This type of hip replacement, called hemiarthroplasty, only addressed the problem of the arthritic femoral head (the ball). The diseased acetabulum (hip socket) was not replaced. The prosthesis consisted of a metal stem which was placed into the marrow cavity of the femur, connected in one piece with a metal ball which fit into the hip socket. While very popular in the 1950s, results remained

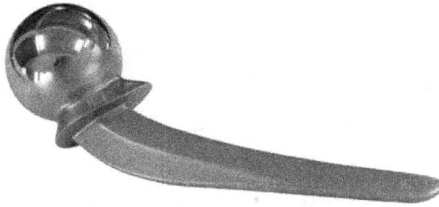

Fig. 1. Thompson.

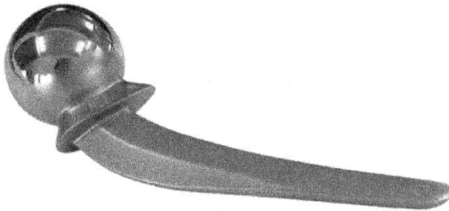

Fig. 2. Moore.

unpredictable and arthritic destruction of the socket persisted. In addition, there was no truly effective method of securing the component to the bone. Large numbers of patients developed pain because of this loosening of the implant. The desired result was still not achieved.

Although the Frenchman Pierre Delbet was the first to use a rubber femoral prosthesis in 1919, a lot of attention for early prostheses was garnered by two fellow countrymen of his: Robert and Jean Judet[6] (see Fig. 3). As early as 1938, they attempted to use an acrylic material to replace arthritic hip surfaces. This acrylic provided a smooth surface, but unfortunately tended to come loose.

The idea did lead Dr. Edwarc J. Haboush from the Hospital for Joint Diseases in New York City to utilize a "fast-setting dental acrylic" to actually glue the prosthesis to the bone. A new era in fixation techniques had begun.

In England, a very innovative surgeon, John Charnley[7] was also attempting to solve these ongoing problems. He aggressively pursued effective methods of replacing both the femoral head and acetabulum

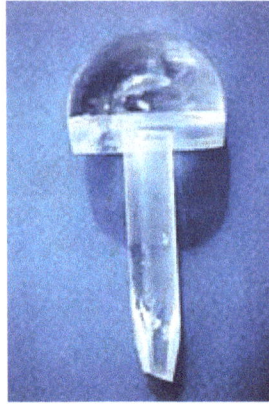

Fig. 3.   Judet.

of the hip. In 1958, he addressed the eroded arthritic socket by replacing it with a Teflon implant. He hoped this would allow for a smooth joint surface to articulate with the metal ball component. When the Teflon did not achieve this goal, he went on to try polyethylene, which worked very well. In order to obtain fixation of this polyethylene socket, as well as the femoral implant to the bone, Charnley borrowed polymethylmethacrylate from the dentists. This substance, known as bone cement, was mixed during the operation and then used as a strong grouting agent to firmly secure the artificial joint to the bone. This was truly the birth of "total hip replacement" (see Fig. 4).

Since that time, many skilled surgeons have improved upon the concepts developed in central England. Methods of fixation and actual cementing techniques are significantly better and refinements in the design of the prosthesis have evolved to more clearly mirror the normal hip joint. Today over 15,000 hip replacements are performed annually in the Netherlands using the principles of a low-friction arthroplasty with a polyethylene socket and metal femoral prosthesis.

The Development of Knee Prostheses

The development of total knee arthroplasty in many ways paralleled that of total hip arthroplasty. The first attempt at total knee

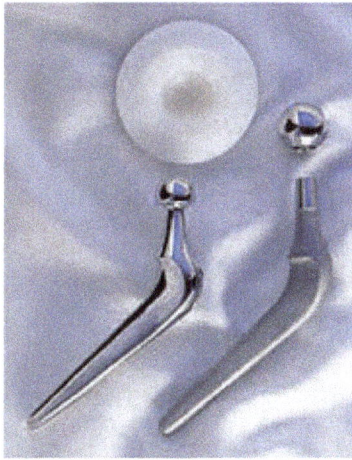

Fig. 4.   Charnley.

arthroplasty was a prosthesis, which was really a hinge fixed to the bones with stems placed into the medullary canals (the hollow marrow cavity). These hinges provided good short-term pain relief, but function was not always great due to the limited range of motion. After a few short years, this prosthesis showed severe problems with loosening and infection and was abandoned. During this same period of time, some surgeons were trying to treat arthritis of the knee with a metal spacer which was placed between the bones of the knee to eliminate the rubbing of irregular surfaces against each other. These implants, the McKeever (1957) and MacIntosh (1958, 1964),[8] achieved some success, but were not predictable, and many patients continued with significant symptoms. Next, surgeons at Massachusetts General Hospital made a prosthesis in the shape of the femoral half of the knee joint. This mold-type arthroplasty helped in relieving symptoms but was not predictable, nor were the results always lasting. These "primitive" replacements evolved from 1940 to 1965.

During the late 1960s, a Canadian orthopedist, Frank Gunston,[9] from Sir John Charnley's Hip Center, developed a metal-on-plastic knee replacement secured to the bone with cement. This was really the first metal and plastic knee, and the first with cement fixation

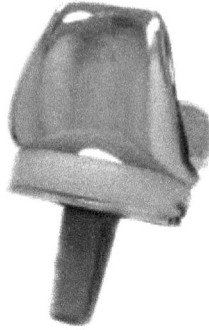

Fig. 5.   A total condylar knee.

(1968) — the era of total knee arthroplasty had begun. In 1972 another Englishman living in New York City, John Insall[10] MD, designed what has become the prototype for current total knee replacements (see Fig. 5). This was a prosthesis made of three components which would resurface all three surfaces of the knee — the femur, tibia and patella (kneecap).

They were each fixed with bone cement and the results were outstanding. This was the first total knee complete with specific instrumentation to help with accurate bone cutting and implantation. Current research on total knee replacement is directed at refining the design to improve patient function. The desire to achieve greater knee motion and strength motivates researchers to further enhance knee replacements so as to be equal to normal knees.

In the last 10 years there has been considerable effort and research focused on trying to further improve the fixation methods of hip and knee arthroplasties. Occasionally it has been found that cement fixation breaks down over time. To this end, implants with textured surfaces that allow bone to grow into them have been developed. Hydroxyapatite-coated implants have demonstrated extensive bone apposition in animal models.[11-13] The osseous interface develops even in the presence of gaps of 1 mm and relative motion of up to 500 μm. Development of implant-bone interfacial strength is due to the biological effects of released calcium and phosphate ions, although surface roughness leads to increased interface strength in the absence of interface gaps. The clinical results at 15 years after total hip replacements have demonstrated that hydroxyapatite-coated femoral stems perform as well as, and possibly better than, other types of cementless devices, with the added benefit of providing a seal against wear debris. The performance of a hydroxyapatite-coated implant depends on coating properties (thickness, porosity, hydroxyapatite content, and crystallinity), implant roughness, and overall design. The most reliable predictor of the performance of a device is success in long-term clinical studies.[14]

Problems We Face

Aseptic Loosening

If the immediate post-operative phase is successful, aseptic loosening is still the main challenge to overcome in long-term follow-up of arthroplasty. The osteolysis leading to loosening of the components was initially linked to the biomechanical properties of bone cement, and it was named "cement disease."[15] Because uncemented procedures did not protect against osteolysis and loosening, investigators searched for other possible causal factors. Metallic ions and particles have been the subject of investigations, but could not explain the osteolysis around Judet hemiprostheses made of acrylic or nylon, or around uncemented all-polyethylene acetabular components. Currently, the most accepted view is that the effects of polyethylene wear particles are the most important cause of failure, although osteolysis has also been observed in prostheses with ceramic-on-ceramic bearings. Another suggested mechanism of failure is quite the opposite of the accepted wear-induced-loosening theory: the loosening-induced wear theory. It states that early (undetected) loss of fixation is the causal factor behind the observations of periprosthetic granulomas and excessive wear, thus reversing the cause and effect. Animal experimental model studies provide support for this possibility, but future investigations are still needed to clarify the role of each possible causal factor.

Wear has been a primary issue in arthroplasty. The wear of the hard surface of the metal (femoral head or condyles) is negligible.[16,17] Therefore, the continued source of the wear and debris problem is polyethylene in the standard metal-on-polyethylene articulation. Plastic deformation or creep should be distinguished from wear. Creep is plastic deformation of the acetabular liner due to loading, without the production of wear debris or particles. This has been termed "bedding in" or "running in" by several authors. The rate of creep decreases over time and becomes negligible after 12–18 months. The wear resistance of polyethylene is affected by sterilization techniques. Until recently, the industry standard for sterilization has been gamma irradiation in air. Gamma irradiation breaks molecular bonds in the long polyethylene chains, giving rise to free radicals. In an oxygen environment, oxygen combines with these free radicals, leading to subsurface oxidation. As oxidation increases, so does fatigue cracking and delamination. Components that have been on the shelf for less than a year before implantation have shown decreased *in vivo* oxidation and better *in vivo* performance.

Septic Loosening: Infection

Total joint replacement has shown to be a highly effective treatment for end-stage arthritis of the major weight-bearing joints, and hip and knee replacements are therefore very common in orthopedic surgery. It is estimated that approximately 1 million hip replacements and 250,000 knee replacements are carried out per year.[18] This number is expected to double between 1999 and 2025 as a result of aging populations worldwide and growing demand for a higher quality of life. Despite the success of joint arthroplasty, complications persist, including aseptic loosening and infection. There are several theories on how deep infections of joint prostheses develop. Most studies on the interaction of the prosthesis with infecting organisms showed that bacteria attach to the device during implantation. Once the bacteria are attached, many encase themselves in a protective biofilm. The bacteria within a biofilm can remain "quietly" on the surface of the prosthesis for a long period of time. However, when environmental influences, such as a decreased host immune function or poor tissue ingrowth around the joint prosthesis, deteriorate, the biofilm bacteria can give rise to a clinical infection (see Fig. 6).

Bacteria isolated from orthopedic infections are frequently *Staphylococcus* species, with Coagulase-negative staphylococci as the predominant ones, while aerobic Gram-negative bacteria cause 10–20% of all deep infections and anaerobic bacteria are responsible for another 10–15%.[19,20] With routine hospital culturing, mostly only one causative organism is found on infected implants, but using more extensive culturing techniques, many infections seem to be polymicrobial.[21,22]

The infection rate of primary joint arthroplasties is estimated nowadays between 1% and 3%.[23,24] This percentage may seem small, but since these joint replacement operations are so common, it is a complication that affects a significant number of patients. Although relatively uncommon, infection remains a devastating complication from the perspective of both the patient and society. Infection is connected to a substantial increase in morbidity, which increases hospital admittance time, and hence adds significant costs to the health care system. At an average cost of $55,000 per treatment of

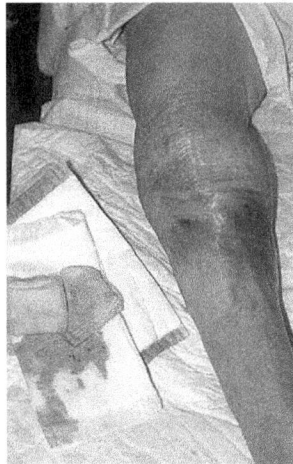

Fig. 6.   An infected total knee replacement.

an infected joint replacement, the costs in the United States alone are about \$250 million for the management of infected replacements,[18] and approximately triple that amount worldwide.

Joint replacement infections will, in general, not clear until the implant is removed, and the patient must then be given antibiotic therapy. This treatment can prolong the patient's hospital stay by weeks and require additional surgery, resulting in high cost for the health care system and increased suffering by the patient. A more convenient way to deal with this problem is to prevent the development of an infectious biofilm on the implant surface.

Prevention of Biomaterial-related Infections in Orthopedic Implants

Polymethylmethacrylate (PMMA) bone cement is a material widely used to anchor prostheses during joint replacement surgery (see Fig. 7). PMMA bone cement was introduced[25] to stabilize metallic hip implants and transfer mechanical loads from the implant to the bone and vice versa. The introduction of **antibiotic-loaded bone**

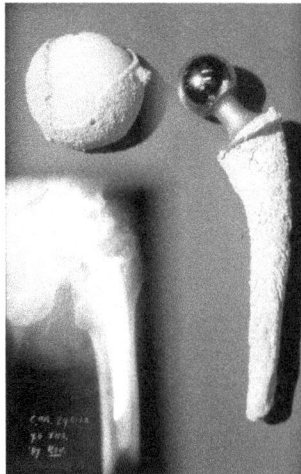

Fig. 7.   Removed total hip replacement that was fixed with bone cement to the patient's bone. Insert: X-ray of the total hip replacement before revision surgery.

cement was meant to establish a decrease of the implant infection rates.[26] The assumption underlying the incorporation of antibiotics in bone cements was that the antibiotic would gradually be released to yield higher local concentrations than can be achieved by systemic therapy.

A study conducted by Buchholz *et al.*[27] between 1972 and 1975 found an infection frequency of 1.6% for total hip replacements using gentamicin-loaded bone cement. In contrast, the frequency of deep infections for hip replacements bone cement without gentamicin was 4.9%. Other authors reported similar results. In fact, in almost every documented study since then, the infection rate of primary joint replacements using antibiotic-loaded bone cement has been significantly lower than when plain bone cements or systemic antibiotics are used.[28–30] Consequently, many surgeons have routinely used antibiotic-loaded bone cement in all primary joint replacements.

Mechanisms of Antibiotic Release from Bone Cements

Bone cements are made up of two primary components (see Table 1): a powder containing copolymers based on the substance polymethylmethacrylate, and a liquid monomer, methylmethacrylate. The powder component consists of beads; the size of these beads varies between 5 and 80 μm and the beads are usually clearly visible in electron micrographs of bone cement samples (see Fig. 8). The powder also contains a starter, benzoyl peroxide, while the liquid contains the initiator, N,N-dimethyl-p-toluidine. Both substances together start the polymerization process and enable a reaction at room temperature. A special radio-opaque agent (zirconium dioxide or barium sulphate) is added to the powder to provide X-ray contrast. The powder component in antibiotic-loaded bone cements contains an antibiotic, such as gentamicin in Palacos R and erythromycin in Simplex P. Cements are loaded with the mechanical safe maximum of 1 g antibiotic base per 40 g powder.

There is now enough evidence that when antibiotic is added to PMMA bone cement it will be released, but the mechanism by which these drugs are released is still under debate. The most accepted

Table 1. Composition of Three Different Antibiotic-loaded Bone Cements, Expressed in Grams, Respectively as Given by the Manufacturer

	Palacos R	CMW 3	Simplex
POWDER			
Poly(methylmethacrylate, stryrene)	—	—	29.51
Poly(methylmethacrylate)	—	—	5.91
Poly(methylacrylate, methyl methacrylate)	33.55	33.55	—
Barium sulphate	—	4.00	4.00
Zirconium dioxide	6.13	—	—
Benzoyl peroxide	0.32	0.76	0.58
Gentamine sulphate	0.84	1.69	—
Erythromycin-gluco heptonate	—	—	0.73
Colistin-methane sulfonate-sodium	—	—	0.24
Chlorophyllin	0.001	—	—
LIQUID			
Methyl methacrylate	18.40	17.45	18.31
N,N-dimethyl-p-toluidine	0.38	0.45	0.48
Chlorophyllin	0.0004	—	—
Hydroquinone	—	25 ppm	0.0015

theory is that antibiotic release is a surface phenomenon and is based on the fact that most of the antibiotic remains trapped within the polymer matrix. PMMA is capable of taking up very small quantities of dissolution fluid into its outermost layers, and this fluid then slowly transports the antibiotic molecules out into the surrounding tissue. Initially, when the infection is still very active, large amounts of antibiotic are released,[31] because it is particularly easily available at the surface of bone cement.

The sustained release of antibiotics from bone cements is largely influenced by the penetration of fluids into the polymer matrix, which requires a certain porosity of the cement[32,33] (see Fig. 8). A point on which all studies have agreed is that the period of maximum antibiotic release is limited to the first few hours or days after implantation.[34] Most, if not all, of the antibiotic is released from the

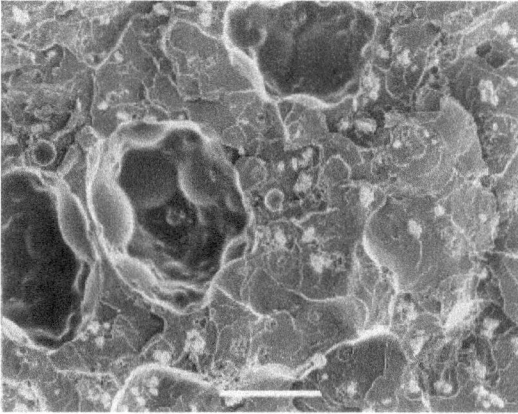

Fig. 8. Scanning electron micrograph showing the matrix of a high-porosity cement (Palamed). The bar represents 100 μm.

(Reprinted from Biomaterials, Van de Belt H, Neut D, Van Horn JR, Van der Mei HC, Uges DRA, Schenk W, Busscher HJ. Surface roughness, porosity and wettability of gentamicin-loaded bone cements and their antibiotic release, 1981–1987, (2000), with permission from Elsevier.)

superficial regions of the cement and fails to be released from the centre.[35,36] In fact, many *in vitro* and *in vivo* studies have shown that only small amounts of the antibiotics incorporated into bone cement are actually released, with a maximum of 15%.[32,37]

The porosity of the polymer matrix depends on air entrapment during stirring of the cement paste and on effects of monomer boiling.[38] In addition, the porosity also depends on the viscosity of the cement. High viscosity cements, e.g. Palacos R, possess a higher porosity than low viscosity cements like CMW 3, because of the greater difficulties encountered by entrapped air bubbles trying to escape the polymer matrix. Baker and Greenham[32] concluded that bone cement with greater porosity would be expected to allow more antibiotic release than cement with less porosity. Therefore, methods of cement preparation that are designed to improve its mechanical properties by decreasing the porosity (such as vacuum mixing) could have deleterious effects on the antibiotic release.

Clinical Aspects of Application of Antibiotic-loaded Bone Cements

A problem encountered in the application of antibiotic-loaded bone cements is the chance of introducing resistant strains by releasing sub-inhibitory antibiotic concentrations for many years. Gentamicin, for instance, has remained detectable in joint fluid aspirations and tissue samples for years after using gentamicin-loaded cement for fixation of a joint prosthesis.[39,36] Of patients with an infected hip, in which the joint replacement was fixed using gentamicin-loaded bone cement, 88% harvested at least one infecting staphylococcal strain resistant to gentamicin.[40] The exact mechanism by which this **antibiotic resistance** evolves is not clear, and different possibilities have been reported, including mutation[41] and selection of already existing resistant variants.[42]

The introduction of antibiotic resistance among infecting bacteria is a great risk in modern medicine and various bacteria have already been described that cannot be eradicated with available antibiotics. The frequency of antibiotic resistance has increased in hospital settings, resulting in therapeutic failures, the use of increasingly costly and toxic antibiotics, extended hospital stays, and increased morbidity, mortality, and health care costs. In 1992, 13,300 hospital patients in the United States died of resistant bacterial infections.[43]

Improvements of Commercially Available Antibiotic-Loaded Bone Cements

Antibiotics considered for incorporation into bone cements should demonstrate a broad antibacterial spectrum, including Gram-positive and Gram-negative species, a sufficient bactericidal activity, low allergy potential, good water solubility to facilitate its release from the bone cement, and, last but not least, chemical and thermal stability.[9] Most of the 18 different antibiotic-loaded bone cements currently available on the European market contain gentamicin.[44] Gentamicin shows a good release from bone cement, has a broad antimicrobial spectrum, and kills bacteria instead of inhibiting their growth. However, several *in vitro* (see Fig. 9) and *in vivo* studies indicated bacterial growth on antibiotic-loaded bone cements,[45–47] and this has stimulated interest in improving the existing gentamicin-loaded bone cements, especially taking into account the increased occurrence of gentamicin-resistant bacteria.

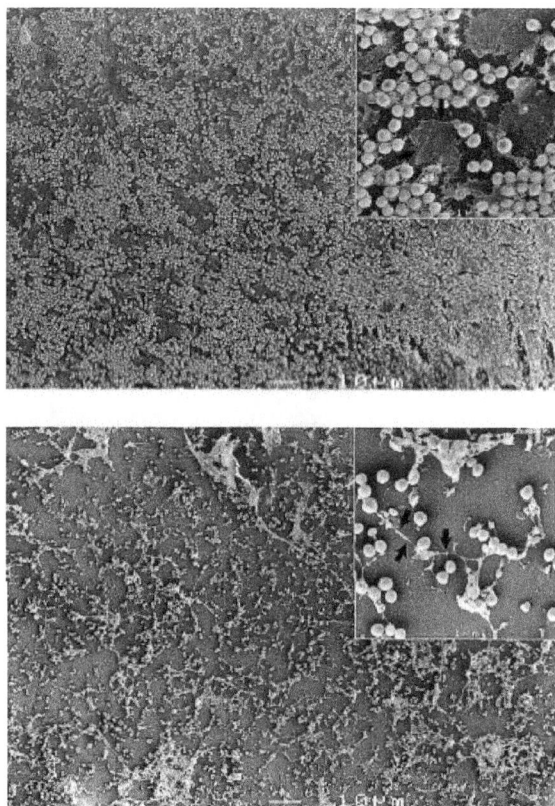

Fig. 9. Scanning electron micrographs of *Staphylococcus aureus* on unloaded (top) and gentamicin-loaded (bottom) bone cement showing the difference in adherence on both type of discs. Slimy films and threads on the antibiotic-loaded cement are indicated by arrows. The bar equals 10 mm for the low magnification micrograph, and 1 mm for the insert.

(Reprinted from ACTA Orthopaedica Scandinavica, Van de Belt H, Neut D, Van Horn JR, Van der Mei HC, Schenk W, Busscher HJ. Gentamicin release from polymethylmethacrylate bone cements and Staphylococcus aureus biofilm formation, 625–629, (2000) with permission from Taylor & Francis.)

Due to this emerging antibiotic resistance there is now a renewed interest in the addition of other antibiotics to bone cements, such as vancomycin and cefuroxime.[48,28] However, from past experience, it is likely that it will only be a matter of time before the bacteria develop a mechanism of resistance to overcome any new antibiotic which is incorporated in bone cement. Therefore, industrial developments include the use of combinations of antibiotics (multi-drug targeting). **Multi-drug targeting** is assumed not only to be more powerful, but also may prevent the emergence of resistant strains through synergistic action of two antibiotics at the same time.[49] In Europe there is already one multi-drug-loaded bone cement commercially available, Copal®, containing gentamicin and clindamycin. A combination of gentamicin and clindamycin in bone cement has a theoretical antimicrobial effect on more than 90% of the bacteria common to infected arthroplasty cases.[44] Moreover, the release of gentamicin seems to be additionally favored by the release of clindamycin in this cement.[44]

Treatment of Chronic Joint Replacement Infections

Once an infection is detected, several options for treatment of infected joint replacements have been established. Which one is used depends on multiple factors, such as type of infection (acute versus chronic), the isolated pathogen and its susceptibility pattern, the fixation of the device, the quality and availability of the bone stock, and the training and experience of the orthopedic surgeon and infectious disease physician. To eradicate chronic prosthesis infection, most authors recommend two-stage revision arthroplasty[42,50] (initial removal and debridement followed by a period of antibiotic treatment, then replacement of the implant). This is recommended because patients with chronic infections are unlikely to respond to antibiotic therapy alone, and moreover, it is impossible to successfully treat a loose prosthesis without removal of the implant. Another treatment option is one-stage revision surgery (removal, debridement and re-implantation all in the same operation). One-stage revision in both the antibiotic-loaded cement group and the unloaded cement group showed an average success rate of 81% and 71%, respectively. Two-stage revision showed higher success rates; 82% in the group with re-implantation without antibiotic-loaded cement, and 93% for the cement loaded with antibiotic.[51] The choice between one-stage or two-stage revision surgery, and the type and duration of antibiotic therapy are mostly dependent on the personal experience of the surgeon. Other treatment options include suppressive antimicrobial therapy, for patients not fit for surgery, and fusion of the joint in late infections.

For successful re-implantation, high concentrations of antibiotic are needed in a localized area to cure the infection. These high concentrations can be achieved through the implantation of chains of **gentamicin-loaded PMMA beads** (see Fig. 10). The gentamicin concentration that can be achieved in this way is much higher than with systemic gentamicin treatment.[52] Usually, the gentamicin-loaded beads are removed after two weeks, and the absence of cultivable bacteria in tissue samples is taken as a sign that the infection is cured and implantation of a new prosthesis can take place.

Despite the advantage of achieving high local antibiotic concentrations of antibiotics with these beads, there are disadvantages, such as limited function of the joint, with the need for bed restriction.

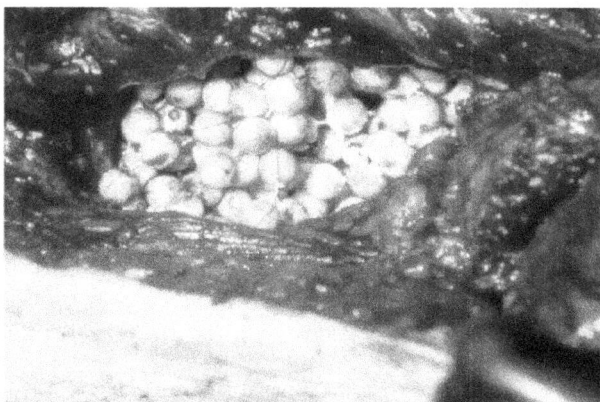

Fig. 10.   Gentamicin-loaded PMMA beads; commercially available in strains of 30 beads.

Instead of implanting gentamicin-loaded PMMA beads, a more-or-less functional **spacer** made of antibiotic-loaded bone cement can be used. The use of differently shaped temporary spacers has proven to be an effective technique for the treatment of infected hip and knee replacements.[53,54] Patients treated with a spacer can walk soon after surgery, thereby decreasing the duration of hospital stay and need for care. Other advantages of spacers are the comfort in which patients await the re-implantation surgery and the easier re-implantation.

References

1. Smith-Petersen MN. (1978) The classic: evolution of mould arthroplasty of the hip joint by M.N. Smith-Petersen. *J Bone Joint Surg* 1948;30B:59. *Clin Orthop Relat Res* 5–11.
2. Smith-Petersen MN. (1939) Arthroplasty of the hip. A new method. *J Bone Joint Surg* 21(2):269–88.
3. Gomez PF, Morcuende JA. (2005) Early attempts at hip arthroplasty — 1700s to 1950s. *Iowa Orthop J* 25:25–9.
4. Thompson FR. (1952) Vitallium intramedullary hip prosthesis, preliminary report. *NY State J Med* 52:3011–20.
5. Moore AT, Bohlman HR. (1943) The classic. Metal hip joint. A case report. *Clin Orthop Relat Res* 3–6.
6. Judet J. (1950) The use of an artificial femoral head for arthroplasty of the hip joint. *J Bone Joint Surg Br* 32-B:166–73.
7. Charnley J. (1961) Arthroplasty of the hip. A new operation. *Lancet* 1:1129–32.
8. McKeever. (1985) The classic: Tibial plateau prosthesis. *Clin Orthop Relat Res* 192:3–15.
9. Gunston FH, MacKenzie RJ. (1976) Complications of plycentric knee arthroplasty. *Clin Orthop Relat Res* 120:11–17.
10. Insall JN. WP. (1979) The total condylar knee prosthesis. *J Bone Joint Surg* 61a:173–80.
11. Geesink RGT, De Groot K, Klein CPAT. (1987) Hip implants with hydroxylapatite coatings. *Acta Orthop Scand* 58(6):731.
12. Geesink RGT, De Groot K. (1987) Biological fixation of apatite-coated protheses. *Acta Orthop Scand* 58(2):203.
13. Geesink RGT. (1989) Experimental and clinical-experience with hydroxyapatite-coated hip implants. *Orthopedics* 12(9):1239–42.
14. Soderman PMHHP. (2000) Outcome after total hip arthroplasty: Part I. General health evaluation in relation to definition of failure in the Swedish National Total Hip Arthoplasty register. *Acta Orthop Scand* 71:354–9.

15. Jones LC. (1987) Cement disease. *Clin Orthop Relat Res* 192–206.
16. Saikko VO. (1993) Wear of polyethylene acetabular cups against alumina femoral heads. 5 prostheses compared in a hip simulator for 35 million walking cycles. *Acta Orthop Scand* **64**:507–12.
17. Willert HGBHBG. (1990) Osteolysis in alloarthroplasty of the hip. The role of ultra-high molecular weight polyethylene wear particles. *Clin Orthop Relat Res* 95–107.
18. Sculco TP. (1995) The economic impact of infected joint arthroplasty. *Orthopedics* **18**:871–3.
19. Fitzgerald RH Jr. (1995) Infected total hip arthroplasty: diagnosis and treatment. *J Am Acad Orthop Surg* **3**:249–62.
20. Garvin KL, Hinrichs SH, Urban JA. (1999) Emerging antibiotic-resistant bacteria. Their treatment in total joint arthroplasty. *Clin Orthop* **369**:110–23.
21. Neut D, Van Horn JR, Van Kooten TG, *et al.* (2003) Detection of biomaterial-associated infections in orthopaedic joint implants. *Clin Orthop* **413**:261–8.
22. Tunney MM, Patrick S, Gorman SP, *et al.* (1998) Improved detection of infection in hip replacements: a currently underestimated problem. *J Bone Joint Surg*, **80B**:568–72.
23. Antti-Poika I, Josefsson G, Konttinen Y, *et al.* (1990) Hip arthroplasty infection. Current concepts. *Acta Orthop Scand* **61**:163–9.
24. Harris WH, Sledge CB. (1990) Total hip and total knee replacement (part II). *N Engl J Med* **323**:801–7.
25. Charnley J. (1970) The reaction of bone to self-curing acrylic cement. A long-term histological study in man. *J Bone Joint Surg Br* **52**:340–53.
26. Buchholz HW, Engelbrecht H. (1970) Über die Depotwirkung einiger Antibiotica bei Vermischung mit dem Kunstharz Palacos. *Chirurg* **40**:511–5.
27. Buchholz HW, Elson RA, Heinert K. (1984) Antibiotic-loaded acrylic cement: current concepts. *Clin Orthop* **190**:96–108.
28. Chiu FY, Chen CM, Lin CF, Lo WH. (2002) Cefuroxime-impregnated cement in primary total knee arthroplasty: a prospective, randomized study of three hundred and forty knees. *J Bone Joint Surg Am* **84**:759–62.
29. Espehaug B, Engesaeter LB, Vollset SE, *et al.* (1997) Antibiotic prophylaxis in total hip arthroplasty. Review of 10,905 primary cemented total hip replacements reported to the Norwegian arthroplasty register, 1987 to 1995. *J Bone Joint Surg Br* **79**:590–5.
30. Josefsson G, Gudmundsson G, Kolmert L, Wijkstrom S. (1990) Prophylaxis with systemic antibiotics versus gentamicin bone cement in total hip arthroplasty. A five-year survey of 1688 hips. *Clin Orthop* **253**:173–8.
31. Van de Belt H, Neut D, Van Horn JR, *et al.* (2000) Surface roughness, porosity and wettability of gentamicin-loaded bone cements and their antibiotic release. *Biomaterials* **21**:1981–7.

32. Baker AS, Greenham LW. (1988) Release of gentamicin from acrylic bone cement. *J Bone Joint Surg Am* **70**:1551–7.
33. Kuechle DK, Landon GC, Musher DM, Noble PC. (1991) Elution of vancomycin, daptomycin and amikacin from acrylic bone cement. *Clin Orthop* **264**:302–8.
34. Trippel SB. Antibiotic-impregnated cement in total joint arthroplasty. *J Bone Joint Surg Am* **68**:1297–1302.
35. Schurman DJ, Trindale C, Hirschman HP, *et al.* (1978) Antibiotic-loaded acrylic bone cement composites. *J Bone Joint Surg Am* **60**:978–84.
36. Wahlig H, Dingeldein E. (1980) Antibiotics and bone cements. Experimental and clinical long-term observations. *Acta Orthop Scand* **51**:49–56.
37. Törholm C, Lidgren L, Lindberg L, Kahlmeter G. (1983) Total hip joint arthroplasty with gentamicin-impregnated cement. A clinical study of gentamicin excretion kinetics. *Clin Orthop* **181**:99–106.
38. Wixson RL, Lautenschlager EP, Novak MA. (1987) Vacuum mixing of acrylic bone cement. *J Arthroplasty* **2**:141–9.
39. Hope PG, Kristinsson KG, Norman P, Elson RA. (1989) Deep infection of cemented total hip arthroplasties caused by coagulase-negative staphylococci. *J Bone Joint Surg Br* **71B**:851–5.
40. Thomes B, Murray P, Bouchier-Hayes D. (2002) Development of resistant strains of *Staphylococcus epidermidis* on gentamicin-loaded bone cement *in vivo*. *J Bone Joint Surg Br* **84B**:758–60.
41. Hendriks JGE, Neut D, Van Horn JR, *et al.* (2005) Bacterial survival in the interfacial gap in gentamicin-loaded acrylic bone cements. *J Bone Joint Surg Br* **87B**:272–6.
42. Neu HC. (1992) The crisis in antibiotic resistance. *Science* **257**:1064–73.
43. Kühn KD. (2000) *Bone Cements. Up-to-date-comparison of Physical and Chemical Properties of Commercial Materials.* Springer-Verlag Berlin Heidelberg, pp. 194–257.
44. Kendall RW, Duncan CP, Smith JA, Ngui-Yen JH. (1996) Persistence of bacteria on antibiotic loaded acrylic depots. *Clin Orthop* **329**:273–80.
45. Oga M, Arizono T, Sugioka Y. (1992) Inhibition of bacterial adherence to tobramycin-impregnated PMMA bone cement. *Acta Orthop Scand* **63**:301–4.
46. Van de Belt H, Neut D, Van Horn JR, *et al.* (1999) Antibiotic resistance — to treat or not to treat? *Nature Med* **5**:358–9.
47. Anagnostakos K, Kelm J, Regitz T, *et al.* (2005) *In vitro* evaluation of antibiotic release from and bacteria growth inhibition by antibiotic-loaded acrylic bone cement spacers. *J Biomed Mater Res B Appl Biomater* **72**:373–8.
48. Murray PR, Pfaller MA, Rosenthal KS, Kobayashi G. (1998) *Medical Microbiology*, Mosby-Year Book, Incorporated, Chapter 20: Antibacterial Agents, 3rd ed., pp. 165–8.

49. McDonald DJ, Fitzgerald RH Jr, Ilstrup DM. (1989) Two-stage reconstruction of a total hip arthroplasty because of infection. *J Bone Joint Surg Am* **71**:828–34.
50. Tattevin P, Cremieux AC, Pottier P, *et al.* (1999) Prosthetic joint infection: when can prosthesis salvage be considered? *Clin Infect Dis* **29**:292–5.
51. Garvin KL, Evans BG, Salvati EA, Brause BD. (1994) Palacos gentamicin for the treatment of deep periprosthetic hip infections. *Clin Orthop* **298**:97–105.
52. Wallenkamp GHIM. (1997) Chronic osteomyelitis. *Acta Orthop Scand* **68**:497–506.
53. Booth RE, Lotke PA. (1989) The results of spacer block technique in revision of infected total knee arthroplasty. *Clin Orthop* **248**:57–60.
54. Duncan CP, Beauchamp C. (1993) A temporary antibiotic-loaded joint replacement system for management of complex infections involving the hip. *Orthop Clin North Am* 751–9.

Case 4

Biomaterials for Voice Reconstruction

G.J. Verkerke, J.W. Tack,* I.F. Herrmann,†
H.F. Mahieu,‡ B.F.A.M. van der Laan§ and
H.K. Schutte**

*A laryngectomy has severe consequences for the patient's quality of
life. The voice becomes low-pitched, nasal functions are lost and
the inevitable visible tracheostoma can be the source of mental
problems. An artificial larynx could solve all of these problems.
However, the function of the larynx is complex. Whether such a
device can be made is questionable and will be discussed. It is
important to realize which functions have to be restored and which
solutions for those functions are available.*

*Department of BioMedical Engineering, University Medical Center Groningen,
University of Groningen, A. Deusinglaan 1, 9713 AV Groningen, The Netherlands.
†Department of Otorhinolaryngology, European Hospital, Via Portuense 700, 00149,
Rome, Italy.
‡Department of Otorhinolaryngology, Vrije University Amsterdam, De Boelelaan
1117, 1081 HV Amsterdam, The Netherlands.
§Department of Otorhinolaryngology, University Medical Center Groningen,
Hanzeplein 1, 9713 GZ Groningen, The Netherlands.

Introduction

The larynx is a fascinating organ; it separates the digestive tract from the respiratory tract, while its distinctive cartilages with joint-like connections provide the means for accurate adjustments to the vocal folds for voice production.

Laryngeal cancer is the most common cancer in the head and neck region. In the Netherlands, for most laryngeal tumors, radiotherapy is the primary choice of treatment, with good results related to tumor response and quality of voice. In patients suffering from high-stage disease or recurrent laryngeal cancer after radiotherapy, a total laryngectomy is the surgical procedure of choice. This mutilating operation influences the quality of life of patients in several ways. The esophagus and trachea are separated as a result of the laryngectomy, after which the patients are required to breathe through a surgically created tracheostoma (see Fig. 1). The loss of voice, due to surgical resection of the larynx, including its vocal folds, is considered to be the most disabling consequence of a total laryngectomy. Therefore, adequate voice rehabilitation is of utmost importance after a total laryngectomy.

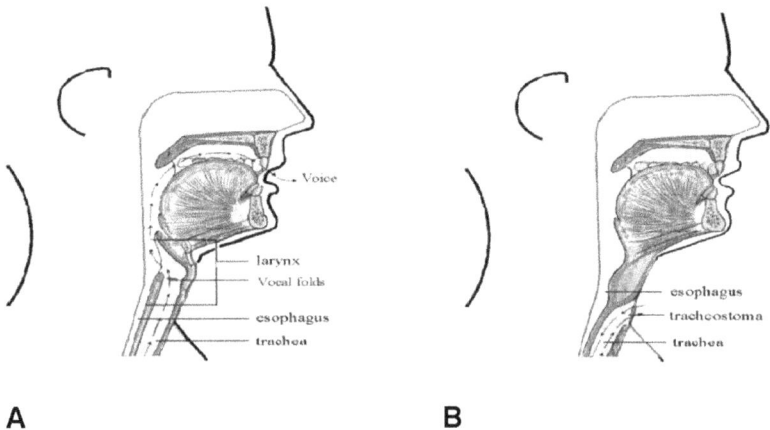

A   **B**

Fig. 1.   Schematic presentation of the oropharyngeal anatomy of a patient before (**A**) and after (**B**) total laryngectomy.

Voice Rehabilitation

There is a colorful history of pioneering events and efforts made by doctors and scientists to create an artificial voice source. Even before the first laryngectomy performed by Billroth in 1873, Czermak reported in 1859 on the design of an artificial voice source for a tracheotomized girl.[1] In his design, the sound was produced by a pneumatically driven metal reed. This reed was housed in a tube leading expiratory air from the tracheostoma to the mouth. A similar metal reed was used as a voice source in a medical implant connecting the tracheostoma and the pharynx. This device was developed by Leiter and Gussenbauer for the first laryngectomy patient, and the design was later modified by others.[2] Besides the pneumatic sound sources, further developments in voice rehabilitation concerned electrically driven sound sources, applied externally or internal. These sound sources all share the same major disadvantage: the resulting voice sounds mechanical and monotonous. A more detailed historical overview of the prototype development for voice rehabilitation is described by various authors, e.g. Lebrun,[2] and Blom.[3]

We will focus now on the current state of voice rehabilitation research. The shunt valve assisted tracheo-esophageal (TE) voice was introduced in 1980 and is currently the most widely used technique. After the surgical operation a one-way shunt valve is placed between the trachea and the esophagus, allowing a flow of air from the lungs into the esophagus when the tracheostoma is closed-off, while food and liquids are prevented from entering the trachea. These valves, such as the ones shown in Fig. 3, are made of silicone rubber and are often called "voice prostheses" in the literature, although they do not actually produce a voice. The sound source is produced by vibrations of remaining muscular structures and mucosa (the pharyngo-esophageal segment) under influence of a passing flow of air.

In this way, most laryngectomized patients can regain an audible voice. Nowadays, this tracheoesophageal shunt speech (see Fig. 2) is considered to be standard in voice rehabilitation.[34]

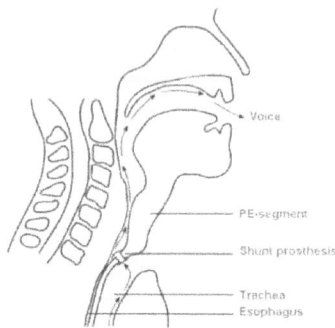

Fig. 2.   Schematic presentation of post-laryngectomy tracheoesophageal speech with a shunt valve inserted into the tracheoesophageal fistula.

Shunt Valves

Since Blom and Singer introduced their duckbill shunt valve in 1979, several types of tracheoesophageal shunt valves have been developed, each with their own valve mechanism design. Nowadays, in the Netherlands, indwelling devices such as the Provox®II and the Groningen button are commonly used.[4] The Groningen button is made of implant-grade silicone rubber and consists of a shaft with two flanges, with a circular slit in the hat of the esophageal flange functioning as a one-way valve. In the Groningen Low Resistance the circular slit is 145° and in the Groningen Ultra Low Resistance the slit is prolonged to 200°. The Provox®II shunt valve is also a biflanged device made of medical-grade silicone rubber. Its hinged valve is molded into one piece with the shaft and is supported by a radiopaque, fluoroplastic ring, which is fastened to the shaft of the prosthesis (see Fig. 3).

Biofilm Formation and Shunt Valves

Biofilms are defined as matrix-enclosed bacterial populations adherent to each other and/or to surfaces. Biofilm formation on shunt valves starts developing from the time the shunt valve is placed into the fistula, as the neopharynx is a non-sterile environment. The

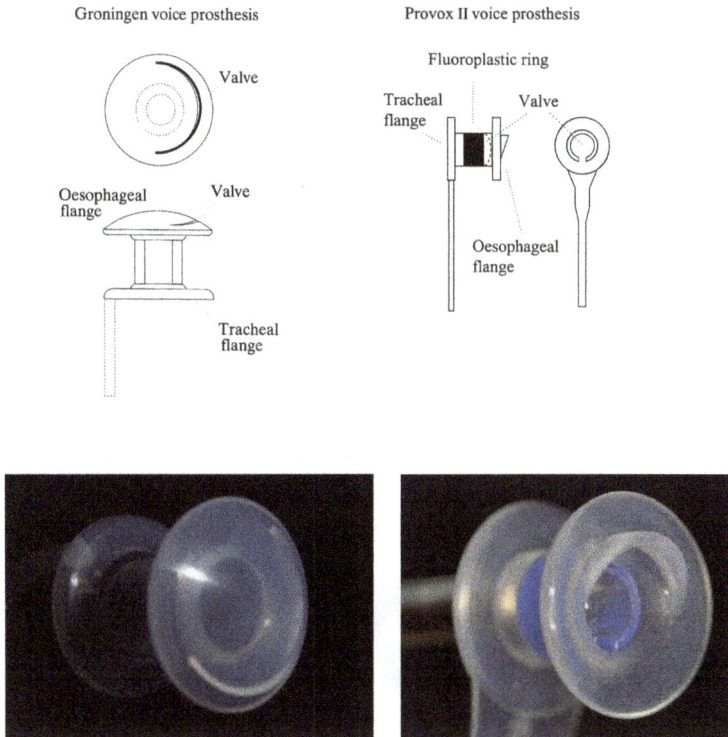

Fig. 3. Schematic presentation and pictures of the Groningen voice prosthesis (*left*) and Provox®II (*right*).

biofilm found on shunt valve is a mixed biofilm consisting of both bacteria and yeast.[5] The organisms found in the shunt valve biofilm are a result of the local oropharyngeal flora and the various components of daily food intake. As a consequence, the composition of the biofilm will differ from person to person.[6] The build-up of a biofilm is a result of adhesive interactions between bacteria and yeast.[7] Bacteria stimulate yeast to adhere to the silicone rubber surface of shunt valves and produce extracellular polymeric substances (EPS) to glue the biofilm into a massive structure. By this mode of growth the biofilm protects itself against antibiotic and antimycotic interventions.[5,8]

Lifetime

The major drawback of shunt valve rehabilitation is the limited lifetime of the shunt valve. Deterioration of the silicone rubber of the valve system by different bacterial and yeast species organized in the form of a biofilm will result in internal leakage or increased airflow resistance, impeding speech, respiration and swallowing.[6,9] Visualization of biofilm architecture shows a large variety in biofilm formation, with an increase of the biofilm thickness and yeasts deteriorated into the silicone rubber in time (see Fig. 4).[10] Therefore, the prostheses need to be replaced on average every 3–4 months.[4,33] However, some patients require more frequent replacements, with intervals of 1–2 weeks. Frequent replacement is harmful to the tracheoesophageal fistula and is uncomfortable for the patient. Keeping

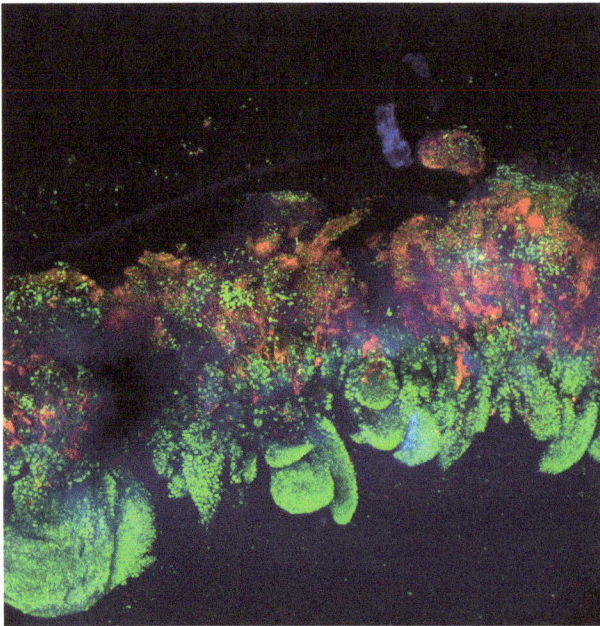

Fig. 4.   Biofilm on top of a ten weeks old Provox®2 silicone rubber shunt prosthesis: Visualization of biofilm architecture by Fluorescence *in situ* Hybridization and Confocal Laser Scanning Microscopy. Red: bacteria, Green: yeasts ingrowth in silicone rubber, Blue: mucus.

all these aspects in mind, it is clear that it is important for the patients' quality of life to prolong the *in situ* lifetime of the tracheoesophageal shunt valve. Extension of the *in situ* lifetime can be achieved with several approaches, for example, by prevention or reduction of the biofilm formation.

Prevention of Biofilm Formation

A biofilm protects itself against antibiotic and antimycotic interventions through its composition. The extracellular polymeric substances (EPS), or slime-embedding organisms, are mainly held responsible for the lack of influence of antibiotics and antimycotics in biofilm-related infections. *In vitro* experiments by Schwandt *et al.* demonstrated that biofilm formation on shunt valves is reduced in an artificial throat by the use of mucolytics, such as N-acetylcysteine.[11] Oosterhof *et al.* stated that mucolytics not only inhibit bacterial growth, but also disrupt the integrity of the biofilm by reducing EPS formation, resulting in a reduction of airflow resistance of shunt valves *in vitro*.[12] As microbial resistance is an increasing problem, the need to explore products other than antibiotics or antimycotics will be an important issue. For this reason, the interest in alternative products such as probiotics has renewed. Free *et al.* have mentioned a reduction of bacteria and yeast in an existing biofilm by certain dairy products investigated in an artificial throat model.[13,14] Schwandt *et al.* demonstrated that there is a positive effect of diary products on biofilm formation in the artificial throat model, and on the lifetime of Provox®II shunt valves *in vitro* and *in vivo*.[11,15] As stated before, biofilm offers an effective protection against antimicrobials and probiotics, therefore preventive measures seem a better way to deal with a biofilm.[16] Prevention of biofilm formation can be achieved by optimizing the silicone rubber manufacturing process or by the use of a coating with antibacterial properties.[17] Oosterhof *et al.* studied the effect of Quaternary Ammonium Silane (QAS) coatings on biofilm formation.[18] The QAS coating seemed to have an inhibiting effect on the formation and ingrowth of biofilm on the shunt valve in *in vitro* experiments. The effect of a super-smooth silicone rubber on biofilm formation is still under investigation (manuscripts in preparation). Finally button design can influence the function and lifetime of the shunt valve.[19] Biomedical engineering of the shunt prosthesis architecture can help the patient by increasing product lifetime and producing a better voice, resulting in a better quality of life.

Voice Production

In a healthy person, the voice is produced through the vibrations of the vocal folds. By the periodical opening and closing of these vocal folds a constant flow of air from the lungs is frequency-modulated. The resulting sound pressure waves set the air in the vocal tract into vibration. The connection of the larynx with this vocal tract, which acts as a resonator, is what makes speech possible. For the pronunciation of the different vowels during speech the shape of the vocal tract changes primarily by movements of the tongue, palate, lower jaw, and lips, thereby resonating specific frequencies available in the harmonically rich voice source.

When the total larynx has to be removed, e.g. due to advanced laryngeal carcinoma, the patient also loses the ability to produce voice in a natural way.

The Substitute Voice Source

Some laryngectomized patients are unable to produce a voice of sufficient quality. Furthermore, the disadvantage of the TE voice is that it usually has a low fundamental frequency (low pitch), which presents a problem, especially for female laryngectomized patients. To overcome these problems, in the past few years efforts have been made to develop a so-called voice-producing element (VPE) that can be introduced into the TE shunt valve (see Fig. 5).

The vocal folds vibrate by a complex co-operation of aerodynamic forces and exerted muscle tensions. Only the aerodynamic forces are available for a substitute voice source placed inside a TE shunt valve. Still, it is necessary to provide the means for intonation

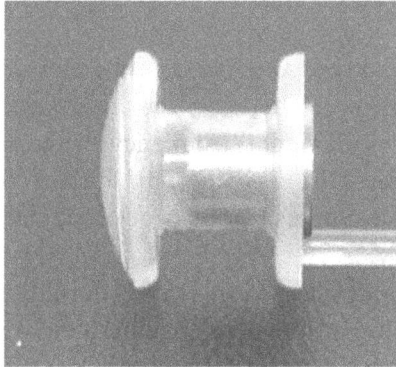

Fig. 5. Groningen Button-type shunt valve, with the valve on the left (esophageal) side and a voice-producing element prototype inserted at the right (tracheal) side.

during laryngectomized patients' speech. Therefore, the fundamental frequency of the sound produced with the VPE should increase by an increase in driving lung pressure. The level of the fundamental frequency should be appropriate for producing a male (mean 120 Hz) or female (mean 210 Hz) voice, while the effort required to produce the voice in terms of driving lung pressure (approximately 0.2–1.5 kPa) and airflow rate (approximately 45–350 ml/s) should be within physiological limits. Furthermore, for a normal intonation pattern a frequency variation of about 7 semitones (~50%) is required, while the voice should have proper audibility when the sound pressure level ranges from 60 to 80 dB, measured at a distance of 30 cm from the mouth.

Sound Generators

Different sound generating principles can be realized as a VPE to create the substitute voice source. Basically, these devices produce sound by mechanical vibrations of an elastic airway constriction, which periodically closes off the airway as a result of aerodynamic forces. Several concepts and prototypes that have been investigated will be reviewed here, also indicating their strengths and weaknesses.

Metal Reed

In the past, the metal reed was the sound generator most frequently used to replace the voice. The reason for this is probably the relative ease of tuning the fundamental frequency of the sound produced to the frequency desired during the design. Furthermore, a clear sound containing strong harmonics can be produced, and the sound usually has a good intensity.

Hagen *et al.*[20] and Herrmann *et al.*[21] developed and tested VPE prototypes containing an inwards-striking metal reed, such as found in a mouth-organ (see Fig. 6a). These prototypes, which also contained a valve, were manufactured by the company ESKA Implants GmbH (Lübeck, Germany). Using this device, patients were able to produce clear voiced sounds, with suitable fundamental frequencies. However, this fundamental frequency was invariable, leading to a monotonous voice. Furthermore, the element appeared to be sensitive to blockage by tracheal secretions.

Siren

The siren, a rotating disk with holes, periodically cuts off airflow so that pulses of air are produced. The characteristic feature of the siren is the favorably direct dependency of the fundamental frequency on

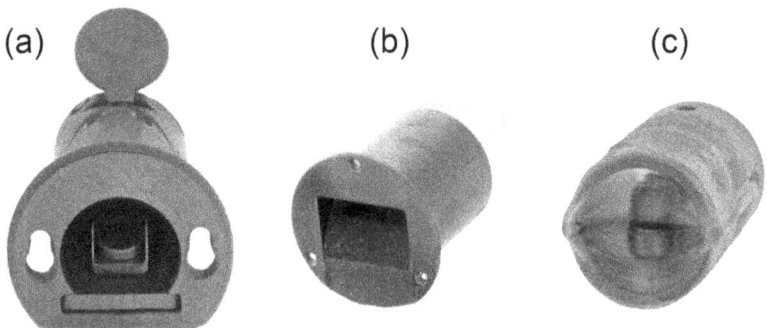

Fig. 6.   Photograph of three voice-producing element prototypes, containing different pneumatically driven sound generators; (a) metal reed, (b) silicone rubber lip, (c) polyurethane membranes.

the driving air pressure, as the frequency increases with increasing rotational speed. The level of the frequency mainly depends on the number of holes applied. The rotating part is also the weakness of this concept, since mucus from the trachea will almost immediately block the disc.

Silicone Rubber Lip

An elastic airway constriction made of a flexible rubber can be designed in many different shapes, and made out of different materials. In comparison with metal reeds, the advantage of the flexible material is usually a more natural sound, while, because of nonlinear dynamics, the fundamental frequency is dependent on the magnitude of the aerodynamic forces. The simplest shape is that of a single lip, fixed on one side of its extremities.

De Vries *et al.*[22] developed a VPE consisting of an outwards-striking silicone rubber lip placed in a square housing (see Fig. 6b). In rest, the lip is bent and presses against the upper wall. Under influence of a flow of air the lip starts to vibrate. Although the sound characteristics are considered suitable for producing voice, in clinical tests it was observed that the functioning of the silicone rubber lip was sensitive to the mucus that entered the prototype[23] and that the lip sometimes stuck to the interior of its housing.

Polyurethane Membranes

To overcome the negative influences of the tracheal mucus, a membrane-based VPE is under development at the Department of BioMedical Engineering, University Medical Center Groningen (Groningen, The Netherlands).[24] This sound generator comprises two weighted polyurethane membranes placed parallel to each other inside a circular housing (see Fig. 6c). This membrane concept is expected to be less sensitive to blockage by mucus, since the exhaling air has to pass the lumen between the membranes, thus removing the mucus. Moreover, the membranes can be pushed away from each other to create a larger through-flow opening for the passing mucus, while afterwards the membranes will always return to their initial position.

In the current state, the prototypes have sound characteristics that are suitable for replacing the female voice.[35] Preliminary clinical tests showed no mucosal influences; the substitute voice *in situ* functioned well and clearly improved the quality of speech.

Future Voice Rehabilitation

Laryngectomy as a treatment of laryngeal cancer is very mutilating, leaving the patient with a low-pitched and sometimes bad-quality voice, a tracheostoma and an inaccessible nasal function. To improve voice quality a voice-producing prosthesis could be applied. To avoid a stoma and restore nasal function, four approaches are possible:

1) *A partial laryngectomy* can be performed to spare the vocal folds and epiglottis.[25] However, this is only possible when the tumor is not widespread.

2) *A passage from trachea to esophagus* and an epiglottis powered by gravity and inertia of food and fluid, sometimes assisted by muscle contraction can be made surgically.[26] However, prevention of aspiration is not guaranteed. Also, voice restoration is difficult.

3) *A larynx transplantation* can be performed.[27] Disadvantages are the limited availability of donor organs, the difficulty in realizing reinnervation, and the lifelong usage of immunosuppressive drugs, increasing the risk of metastasis.[28]

4) *An artificial larynx* can be implanted. Whereas in organs like the heart, kidney, joints, lungs and liver artificial organs and/or organ transplantation are already feasible, larynx replacement is still lacking. Several attempts have been made since the first laryngectomy in 1866,[29] but they have all been unsuccessful, so this option is not realistic at the moment. However, new developments have led to techniques that could be used for an artificial larynx.

Artificial Larynx

The voice-producing prosthesis, as described on page 201, could be used as a high-quality artificial sound source. A tracheostoma valve could be applied as a selection mechanism between breathing and speaking. Recently, two new tracheostoma valves have been developed that require fewer adjustments than previous ones and are less sensitive to phlegm adhesion. The first one, the Adeva Window®[30], is equipped with a cough valve that prevents manual removal of the tracheostoma valve during coughing. The second system is based on closure by inhalation.[31] Coughing is possible, and the rotating valve mechanism allows smooth walls that decrease mucus and phlegm adhesion.

A tissue connector,[32] could serve as an anchoring place for the artificial larynx. New biomaterials or coatings that are developed for shunt valves[17,18] could be used to prevent biofilm adhesion. A valve system, activated by memory metal wires, could prevent aspiration. This system has to consist of a valve mechanism, an actuator to move the valve, an energy source for the actuator and a control signal that initiates closing and opening. Muscle activity is a suitable control mechanism. To trigger closing, the EMG-signal of a suitable muscle could be used. For opening, the EMG-signal of another muscle (involved in inhalation) could be used. To activate the valve mechanism, memory metal wires can be used. Heating them by an electric current causes a considerable change in length (up to 8%), which can be used to open or close the valve. The memory metal wires work reliable in many applications and the small dimensions make them perfect to sit in the restricted space of the artificial larynx. A battery can be used as power supply, recharged via an existing transcutaneous energy transmission system.

Combining all components will result in an artificial larynx. A first impression is given in Fig. 7. The main problem is the feasibility of the valve system control. Knowledge of the effect of deglutition, aspiration and vomiting on the muscles that are involved in those processes and on timing and sequence of these muscles is still too limited. Another problem in developing an artificial larynx is to achieve absolute "failsafeness."

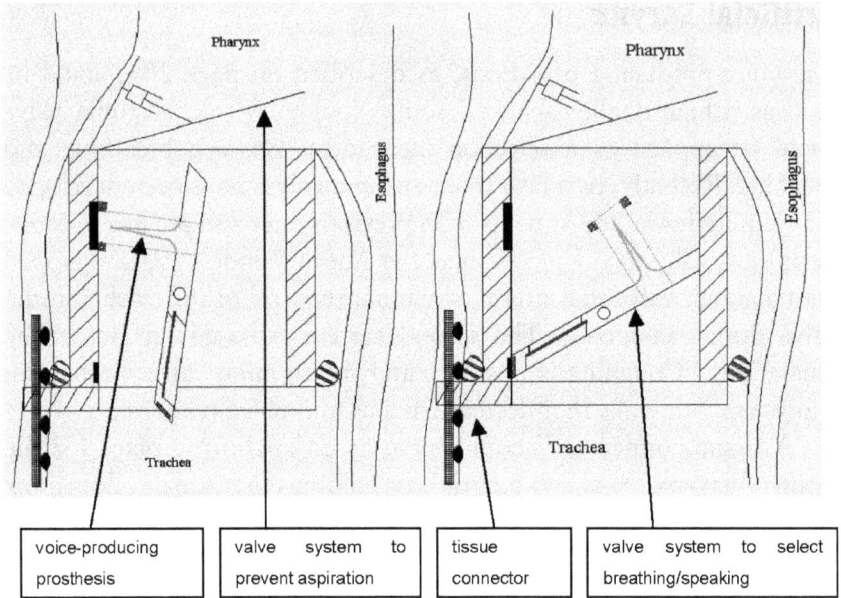

| voice-producing prosthesis | valve system to prevent aspiration | tissue connector | valve system to select breathing/speaking |

Fig. 7. Impression of an artificial larynx in breathing position (*left*) and speaking position (*right*).

Preventing aspiration is the most difficult function to achieve.

Any blockage of respiration will be fatal for the patient. Also, maintenance of the artificial larynx to remove phlegm, mucus and saliva must be avoided as much as possible, since it is very difficult to approach and clean an artificial larynx.

Most of the technology required for the development of an artificial larynx is available. However, sufficient knowledge of proper control signals for the valve system is lacking. "Failsafeness" and insusceptibility for phlegm, mucus and saliva are requirements that will be very difficult to fulfill. Thus realization of an artificial larynx is not expected in the near future.

The "failsafeness" of an artificial larynx is its most difficult requirement.

Acknowledgments

We thank all participants who are involved in the described research projects; participants of the Department of Biomedical Engineering, the Department of Otorhinolaryngology/Head and Neck Surgery, University Medical Center Groningen, University of Groningen, and all participants of Eureka project EU-723 "Artificial larynx" and EU-2614 "Newvoice" for their contribution.

References

1. Czermak J. (1859) *Über die sprache bei luftdichter Verschliessung des Kehlkopfes. Sitzungsberichte der Akademie der Wissenschaften in Wien Mathematischnaturwissenschaftliche Klasse* 35:65–72.
2. Lebrun Y. (1973) *The Artificial Larynx.* Zwets & Zeitlinger BV, Amsterdam.
3. Blom ED. (1978) The artificial larynx: past and present. In: Salmon SJ, Goldstein LP (eds.), *The Artificial Larynx Handbook,* Grune & Stratton, New York, pp. 57–86.
4. Ackerstaff AH, Hilgers FJ, Meeuwis CA, *et al.* (1999) Multi-institutional assessment of the Provox 2 voice prosthesis. *Arch Otolaryngol Head Neck Surg* 125(2):167–73.
5. Stewart PS, Costerton JW. (2001) Antibiotic resistance of bacteria in biofilms. *Lancet* 358(9276):135–8.
6. Neu TR, Dijk F, Verkerke GJ, *et al.* (1992) Scanning electron microscopy study of biofilms on silicone voice prostheses. *Cells and Materials* 2(3):261–9.
7. Millsap KW, Van der Mei HC, Bos R, Busscher HJ. (1998) Adhesive interactions between medically important yeast and bacteria. *FEMS Microbiol Rev* 21(4):321–36.
8. Van der Mei HC, Free RH, Elving GJ, *et al.* (2000) Effect of probiotic bacteria on prevalence of yeasts in oropharyngeal biofilms on silicone rubber voice prostheses *in vitro. J Med Microbiol* 49(8):713–8.
9. Schwandt LQ, Tjong-Ayong HJ, Van Weissenbruch R, *et al.* (2006) Differences in aerodynamic characteristics of new and dysfunctional Provox((R))2 voice prostheses *in vivo. Eur Arch Otorhinolaryngol* Jan 19;1–6 [Epub ahead of print].
10. Buijssen KJDA, Atema-Smit J, Van der Mei HC, *et al.* Visualization by fluorescence *in situ* hybridization and confocal laser scanning microscopy of biofilm architecture on used voice prostheses. (submitted).
11. Schwandt LQ, Van Weissenbruch R, Stokroos I, *et al.* (2004) Prevention of biofilm formation by dairy products and N-acetylcysteine on voice prostheses in an artificial throat. *Acta Otolaryngol* 124(6):726–31.

12. Oosterhof JJ, Elving GJ, Stokroos I, *et al.* (2003) The influence of antimicrobial peptides and mucolytics on the integrity of biofilms consisting of bacteria and yeasts as affecting voice prosthetic air flow resistances. *Biofouling* 19(6):347–53.

13. Free RH, Busscher HJ, Elving GJ, *et al.* (2001) Biofilm formation on voice prostheses: *in vitro* influence of probiotics. *Ann Otol Rhinol Laryngol* 110(10):946–51.

14. Free RH, Van der Mei HC, Dijk F, *et al.* (2000) Biofilm formation on voice prostheses: influence of dairy products *in vitro*. *Acta Otolaryngol* 120(1):92–9.

15. Schwandt LQ, Van Weissenbruch R, Van der Mei HC, *et al.* (2005) Effect of dairy products on the lifetime of Provox2 voice prostheses *in vitro* and *in vivo*. *Head Neck* 27(6):471–7.

16. Costerton JW, Stewart PS, Greenberg EP. (1999) Bacterial biofilms: a common cause of persistent infections. *Science* 284:1318–22.

17. Gottenbos B, Van der Mei HC, Klatter F, *et al.* (2002) *In vitro* and *in vivo* antimicrobial activity of covalently coupled quaternary ammonium silane coatings on silicone rubber. *Biomaterials* 23:1417–23.

18. Oosterhof JJH, Buijssen KJDA, Busscher HJ, *et al.* (2006) Effects of quaternary ammonium silane coatings on mixed fungal and bacterial, tracheoesophageal shunt prosthetic biofilms. *Appl Microbiol*, accepted for publication.

19. Oosterhof JJ, Van der Mei HC, Busscher HJ, *et al.* (2005) *In vitro* leakage susceptibility of tracheoesophageal shunt prostheses in the absence and presence of a biofilm. *J Biomed Mater Res B Appl Biomater* 73(1):23–8.

20. Hagen R, Berning K, Korn M, Schon F. (1998) Stimmprothesen mit tonerzeugendem Metallzungen-Element — A experimentelle und erste klinische Ergebnisse. [Voice prostheses with sound-producing metal reed element — an experimental study and initial clinical results]. *Laryngorhinootologie* 77(6):312–21.

21. Herrmann IF, Arca Recio S, Algaba J. (1996) A new concept of surgical voice restoration after total laryngectomy: the female voice. *The Second International Symposium on Laryngeal and Tracheal Reconstruction* 263–6.

22. De Vries MP, Van der Plaats A, Van der Torn M, *et al.* (2000) Design and *in vitro* testing of a voice-producing element for laryngectomized patients. *Int J Artif Organs* 23(7):462–72.

23. Van der Torn M, Verdonck-de Leeuw IM, Festen JM, *et al.* (2001) Female-pitched sound-producing voice prostheses — initial experimental and clinical results. *Eur Arch Otorhinolaryngol* 258(8):397–405.

24. Tack JW, Verkerke GJ, Houwen EB van der, *et al.* (2006) Development of a double-membrane sound generator for application in a voice-producing element for laryngectomized patients. *Ann Biomed Eng* 34:1896–1907.

25. Marchese Ragona R, Marioni G, Chiarello G, *et al.* (2005) Supracricoid laryngectomy with cricohyoidopexy for recurrence of early stage glottic carcinoma after irradiation. Long-term oncological and functional results. *Acta Otolaryngol* **125**(1):91–5.

26. Algaba J, Zulueta A, Camacho JJ, *et al.* (1996) Primary tracheoesophageal shunt competent for deglutition. In: Algaba J (ed.), *Surgery and Prosthetic Voice Restoration after Total and Subtotal Laryngectomy*, Elsevier, Amsterdam.

27. Strome M, Stein J, Esclamado R, *et al.* (2001) Laryngeal transplantation and 40 month follow up. *N Engl J Med* **344**(22):1676–9.

28. Genden EM, Urken ML. (2003) Laryngeal and tracheal transplantation: ethical limitations. *Mt Sinai J Med* **70**(3):163–5.

29. Alberti PW. (1975) The evolution of laryngology and laryngectomy in the mid 19th century. *Laryngoscope* **85**:288–98.

30. Geertsema AA, De Vries MP, Schutte HK, *et al.* (1998) *In vitro* measurements of aerodynamic characteristics of an improved tracheostoma valve for laryngectomees. *Eur Arch Otorhinolaryngol* **255**(5):244–9.

31. Geertsema AA, Boonstra CW, Schutte HK, Verkerke GJ. (1999) Design and test of a new tracheostoma valve based on inhalation. *Arch Otol Head Neck Surg* **125**:622–6.

32. Ten Hallers EJO, Marres HAM, Houwen van der EB, *et al.* (2006) Experimental results of the tracheoesophageal tissue connector for improved fixation of shunt valves in laryngectomized patients. *Head Neck* **28**(11):982–9.

33. Van den Hoogen FJ, Oudes MJ, Hombergen G, *et al.* (1996) The Groningen, Nijdam and Provox voice prostheses: a prospective clinical comparison based on 845 replacements. *Acta Otolaryngol* **116**(1):119–24.

34. Blom ED, Hamaker RC. (1996) Tracheoesophageal voice restoration following total laryngectomy. In: Myers EN, Suen J (eds.), *Cancer of the Head and Neck*, WB Saunders Publishers, Philadelphia, pp. 839–52.

35. Tack JW, Rakhorst G, Houwen EB Van der, *et al.* (2007) *In vitro* evaluation of a double-membrane based voice-producing element for laryngectomized patients. *Head Neck* **29**(7): 665–74.

Case 5

Biomaterials in Ophthalmology

S.A. Koopmans* and V.W. Renardel de Lavalette*

In ophthalmology, biomaterials are frequently used in the treatment of various eye diseases. An example of a biomaterial is the intraocular lens. Intraocular lenses are implanted in the eye when the opacified natural lens has been removed by phacoemulsification cataract surgery. The history of intraocular lenses started in 1947 when the first lens was implanted. Initially, many severe complications occurred with intraocular lenses, but due to continuing improvements cataract surgery with intraocular lens implantation is now a very safe and predictable operative procedure. As a result, intraocular lenses are also used for refractive surgery. Biomaterials are also used in the treatment of retinal detachments. Although they are adequate for this goal, there is still room for improvements in these biomaterials.

Introduction

Ophthalmology is a medical discipline which treats diseases that threaten vision. Biomaterials are frequently used during ophthalmic

*Department of Opthalmology, University Medical Center Groningen, Hanzeplein 1, 9713 GZ Groningen, The Netherlands.

surgical procedures and the intraocular lens is probably the most frequently implanted biomaterial. In this chapter the use of intraocular lenses together with cataract surgery is discussed. Also, the use of biomaterials in the posterior eye segment is mentioned. There are more applications of biomaterials in the eye, but we have limited ourselves to these two applications.

Eye Anatomy

Eyelids, Tearfilm

The eye is the most peripheral, and the most accessible, part of the visual system (Fig. 1). Anteriorly, the eyes are covered by the eyelids, which serve to protect the eye. The inner lining of the eyelids is called "conjunctiva." The conjunctiva and the transparent anterior surface of the eye (cornea) are covered by the tearfilm.

Anatomy of the Anterior Eye Segment

The anterior eye segment comprises the cornea, the anterior chamber, the iris, the ciliary body and the lens. The cornea is a transparent tissue which is the first refractive surface of the eye. It is continuous

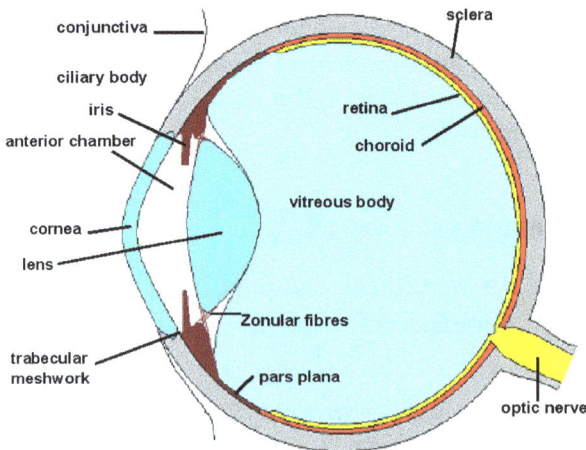

Fig. 1.   Anatomy of the eye.

with the wall of the eye, which is called the sclera. The corneal thickness is about 0.5 mm.[1] The radius of curvature in the center of the cornea is 7.8 mm and its refractive index is 1.376. The optical power is about 43 Diopters. The space between the cornea and the anterior surface of the lens is called the anterior chamber and it is filled with a liquid called aqueous. The anterior chamber depth is about 3 mm from the posterior side of the cornea to the anterior lens surface. The aqueous is produced in the ciliary body. This structure lies at the root of the iris and is continuous with it. The aqueous flows through the pupillary opening and is drained by the trabecular meshwork, situated between the cornea and the iris. The constant production of aqueous together with the drainage by the trabecular meshwork serves to maintain an intraocular pressure, which is usually between 10 and 21 mm Hg. The lens is suspended from the ciliary body via small zonular fibers. It is positioned behind the pupillary opening in the iris and is the second refracting component in the eye. The anterior surface of the lens has a radius of curvature of 11 mm and the posterior surface has a radius of curvature of 5.8 mm at the age of 35 years. At that age, the lens thickness[2] is 3.8 mm. During life, the lens grows, resulting in a slow change in its dimensions and in its optical properties. The optical properties of the cornea usually do not change over time.

The lens is surrounded by a transparent lens capsule with a thickness of approximately 10 μm anteriorly and 4 μm posteriorly. The contents of the lens consist of elongated cells called lens fibers which are arranged in a regular fashion. Towards the center of the lens these fibers are more densely packed than at the periphery of the lens. The outer layers are named lens cortex and the more densely packed inner layers are called the nucleus. The refractive index of the lens contents shows a gradient. At the surface of the lens the refractive index is 1.375 while in the nucleus the refractive index is 1.41.

The optical power of the lens can vary due to contraction of the ciliary muscle in the ciliary body. When the ciliary muscle contracts, the tension on the zonular fibers decreases and the elasticity of the lens capsule causes the lens to take a more spherical shape, increasing its optical power. Relaxation of the ciliary muscle allows elastic fibers in the choroid to pull the lens back in a more flattened state with less optical power.

The process of ciliary muscle contraction, resulting in a change of optical power of the eye, is called accommodation. It enables clear vision of objects nearby. The amplitude of accommodation decreases with age, probably due to increasing sclerosis of the lens contents. Decreased accommodative amplitude causes symptoms such as problems with reading, which usually manifest themselves at the age of 45 years. This is called presbyopia. At the age of 20 years the accommodative amplitude is about 12D, while at the age of 60 years the accommodative amplitude is 0D.

> With aging, the ability of the lens to accommodate is lost.

Anatomy of the Posterior Eye Segment

The tissues behind the lens are called the posterior segment of the eye. Most of the posterior segment is made up of the vitreous, or vitreous body. This is a jelly-like structure mostly made up of water. The retina is the light sensitive layer directly behind the vitreous. Important cells in the retina are the photoreceptor cells, called rods and cones. In these cells, light energy causes a depolarization of the cell membrane, thus creating an electrical signal. Via a retinal network of interneurons, the photoreceptor cells connect to the brain by ganglion cells. These ganglion cells have very long axons which leave the eye at the optic disc and make up the optic nerve. The vitreous, which lies in front of the retina, is attached to the retina at the equator of the eye. Another place of attachment of the vitreous is the optic nerve.

> The retina contains the photoreceptor cells. The vitreous body is in close contact with the retina.

Beneath the retina a highly vascular layer called the choroid is found. Anteriorly, it is continuous with the ciliary body and iris. It serves to provide nutrients to the lower layers of the retina. The outer wall of the eye is the sclera which is continuous anteriorly with the cornea.

Cataracts

With aging, the lens may become opacified. These age-related opacifications gradually increase, leading to a disturbance of vision. Any opacification in the lens is called a cataract. Age-related cataracts occur very frequently and are the leading cause of blindness in the world.[3] In the year 2000, 25 million people were estimated to be bilaterally blind due to cataracts.[4] There are various theories that explain why cataracts develop with aging. These include damage of the lens from ultraviolet radiation, oxidative stress or a build up of sugar in the lens.

The treatment of cataracts is surgical. Cataract extraction is an operation during which the opacified lens (lens = phakos) is removed from the eye. To correct the optical defect (aphakia), which is created with removal of the lens, an artificial lens is usually implanted.

Cataract surgery has a very long history and has developed from a very crude form of surgery into a very safe and predictable procedure that restores sight to visually handicapped patients.[5] As a result of this, the number of cataract surgeries increases each year. In the Netherlands 85,000 cataract surgeries were performed in 2000.[6] Worldwide, more than 6 million intraocular lenses are implanted annually.[7] Nowadays, removal of the lens is usually performed through a technique called phacoemulsification.

> Any opacification of the lens is called a "cataract."

Phacoemulsification Cataract Surgery

The operation begins with anesthesia. For cataract surgery, this can be done with an injection of anesthetic agents around the eye called a retrobulbar or peribulbar block. This paralyzes the eye movements, causing anesthesia and a temporary decrease of vision. An alternative anesthesia method is to apply anesthetizing eyedrops which anesthetize the surface of the eye but leave the eye movements and vision intact. General anesthesia is also possible, but this requires more equipment, time and personnel. As a result of this, the majority of cataract surgeries are performed under local anesthesia in a day-care setting. Pre-operatively, the pupil of the eye is dilated with dilating eyedrops and the eyelids are kept open with a metal eyelid speculum.

To gain access to the lens, an incision is made through the cornea or corneoscleral junction into the anterior chamber (see Fig. 2A). This entrance is made with a flat, 3 mm blade, which creates a self sealing, tunnel-like incision. The anterior chamber is filled with a viscoelastic substance, in order to maintain space between cornea and lens (see Fig. 2B). Usually a solution of sodium-hyaluronate is used. The anterior lens capsule is torn away with forceps in a circular movement so that a round opening is created in the anterior lens capsule (see Fig. 2C). Such circular openings are strong and prevent radial tears of the lens capsule to the lens periphery. Then a phaco emulsification probe is inserted in the eye through the corneal incision and via the anterior chamber into the lens (see Fig. 2D). This phacoemulsification probe allows emulsification of the opacified lens contents with ultrasound energy. The emulsified lens material is aspirated through the lumen of the hollow phacoemulsification needle. At the same time, continuous irrigation of a balanced salt solution in the eye through the phacoemulsification probe keeps the eye pressurized. The lens nucleus is removed with ultrasound energy. The cortex of the lens is relatively soft and is usually removed with another, aspirating hand piece (see Fig. 2E). After removal of the lens contents, the emptied lens capsule, called capsular bag, remains. The anterior chamber is filled with viscoelastic material and an intraocular lens can be implanted in the capsular bag. Since the incision size in the eye is usually around 3 mm, a foldable lens can be implanted which unfolds in the eye (see Figs. 2F, G and H). The alternative is to implant a rigid, non-foldable lens. For this, the incision has to be enlarged to approximately 6 mm. After implantation of the

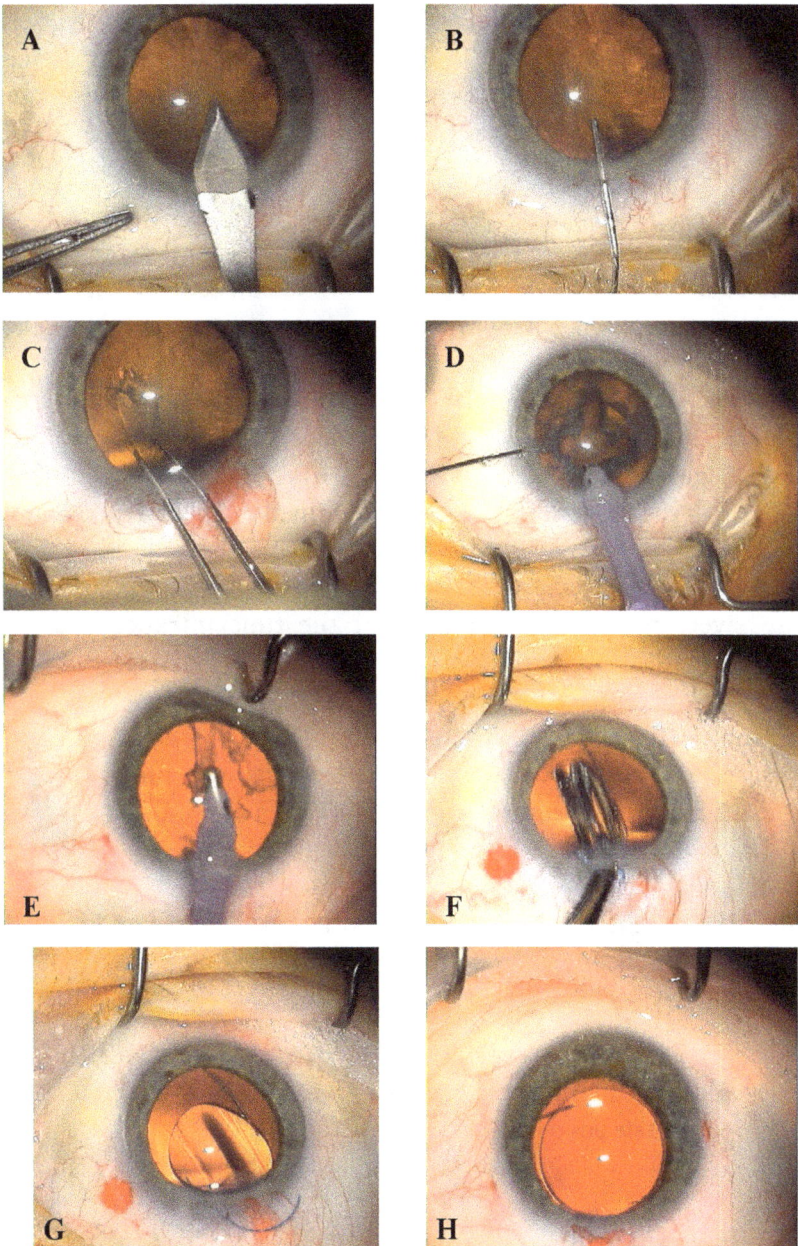

Fig. 2. Removal of the lens by phacoemulsification cataract surgery and implantation of an intraocular lens.

lens, the viscoelastic material is aspirated from the eye and the operation is finished (see Fig. 2H). The incisions usually do not require suturing unless signs of leaking are seen by the surgeon. After narrowing of the pupil, the edges of the lens optic are covered by the iris.

Intraocular Lenses

Intraocular lenses where first used in 1947 to correct aphakia.[7] Before that, the cataractous lens was removed from the eye and the patient was left without a lens (aphakic). To correct the optical defect, the patient was prescribed high plus-powered glasses (+10 to +15 D). Contact lenses could also be used to correct aphakia. High plus-powered glasses limit the visual field of the patient and stereoscopic vision with these glasses can only be obtained after bilateral cataract extraction. Contact lenses do not suffer from these disadvantages, but they can be difficult to handle for elderly people. Also, contact lenses were not widely available at the time intraocular lenses were developed. Implantation of an intraocular lens solves the disadvantages of aphakic glasses and contact lenses. However, the first generations of intraocular lenses created their own specific problems. It has taken several decades before lens manufacturers and eye surgeons have learned how to design and use a safe intraocular lens.[5]

There are three requirements for a safe intraocular lens. First, the lens material has to be transparent and tolerated by the eye. Second, it has to have the right size, shape and power. Third, the lens position has to be secure and safe for the eye.

> The intraocular lens material must be safe for the eye. An intraocular lens must have the right size, shape and power and it must be implanted in a stable, safe position in the eye.

Lens Material

During and directly after the second world war, ophthalmologists observed that fragments from the canopies of the cockpits of combat aircraft which were found in the eyes of the wounded pilots did not cause any harm or inflammation to the eye. The canopies of the cockpits were made of Perspex (Polymethylmethacrylate, or PMMA). This observation lead Dr. Harold Ridley[7] to use PMMA for manufacturing the first intraocular lenses. These first intraocular lenses were implanted in 1949. Although many complications occurred after the first lens implantations, PMMA as a lens material turned out to be successful and it is still used today. About 30 years later, after the development of phacoemulsification, surgeons had the opportunity to remove the cataractous lens through a small, 3 mm incision and a desire for a foldable lens implant material rose. Small incisions in the eye heal faster, cause less inflammation and do not affect the shape of the cornea. The first foldable lens materials were silicones. Later, acrylic materials and hydrogels were developed. Lenses made from foldable materials are folded outside the eye with special folding forceps and then implanted in the eye (see Fig. 2F). Alternatively, they are implanted with an injector system (see Fig. 5). In these systems, the lens folds itself when it is pushed through a narrow injection tip by a plunger. Today, lenses made of PMMA, hydrophobic acrylic and silicone material are implanted most frequently.

> PMMA, silicones and acrylates are used for the manufacturing of intraocular lenses.

Size, Shape and Power

The first intraocular lenses implanted by Ridley were very heavy and dislocated easily from their position behind the iris. The lens power of the first implants was also too high, which resulted in the need for high spectacle corrections. Sterilization was performed by cetrimide, which leached out of the PMMA material in the eye, causing inflammation. Ridley met strong opposition from fellow ophthalmologists, who considered the intraocular lenses as foreign bodies that had to

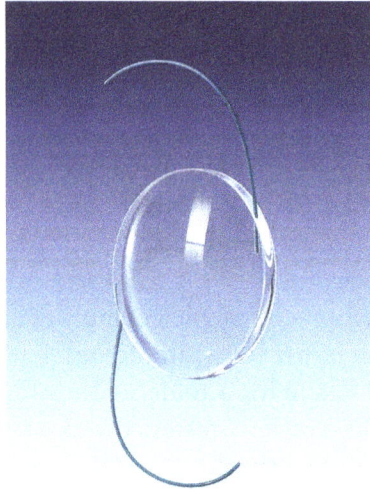

Fig. 3.   Example of an intraocular lens with a circular optic and two J- or C-shaped loops. This lens is implanted behind the iris, in the empty capsular bag.

be taken out of the eye.[7] Due to the strong opposition and a large number of complications, Ridley discontinued the use of intraocular lenses. However, other ophthalmologists continued the development and refinement of intraocular lenses.[5] Nowadays, the most common intraocular lens consists of a 5–6 mm optic, with two J or C shaped flexible loops which result in a diameter of 12–13 mm (see Fig. 3). The optic is usually the thickest part of the lens, with a thickness of 0.5–1.0 mm, depending on the dioptric power. Most lenses are available in a range of 0–30 D in 0.5–1 D steps, and some in an even wider range.

Before surgery, the power of the cornea and the length of the eye are measured (with ultrasound or optical technology) so that with the help of optical calculations an accurate prediction can be made of the lens power that has to be implanted in order to obtain a desired postoperative refraction.

Position and Fixation

The first intraocular lenses were implanted behind the iris because it was felt that this was the natural position for a lens to be. However, when dislocations occurred, surgeons looked for better ways of fixation. In the days of the first lens implantations, the surgical microscope did not exist. This made proper positioning and placement of an intraocular lens much more difficult than today, regardless of the intended lens position. New lenses were developed that were fixated in the anterior chamber, in the chamber angle. This position turned out to be damaging to the cornea after some time, because it resulted in a painful corneal opacification in some patients. Nowadays, intraocular lenses are mostly fixated in the capsular bag. This has proven to be a stable position, where the lens does not do any damage to other ocular structures. A successful alternative method is iris fixation. Here, the lens is attached to the iris with two claw-like structures which pinch the iris tissue (see Fig. 4). This fixation method was developed by Dr. J.G.F. Worst from Groningen, the Netherlands. This fixation method also offers the possibility to place

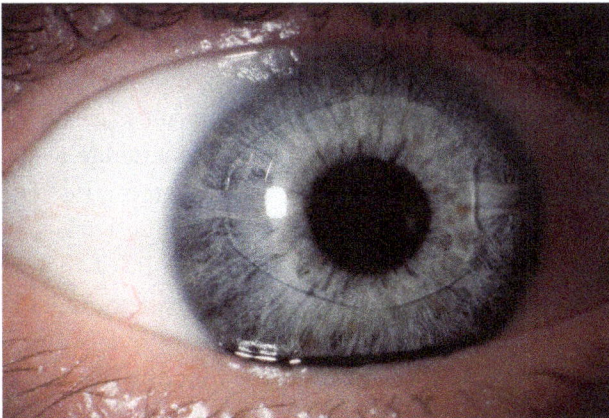

Fig. 4. Example of an Iris-claw lens. The iris is used for fixation. Black nylon sutures are seen in a cross like pattern below the upper eyelid, to close the corneal incision.

an implant lens before the clear, natural lens of a patient, thereby correcting an existing refractive error. This type of surgery is called refractive surgery.

Complications of Intraocular Lens Implantation

Nowadays, removal of a cataract and implantation of an intraocular lens is a very safe, predictable surgical procedure. However, no surgery is free from complications and some of the most important complications are discussed here.

A first complication which can occur after cataract surgery is posterior capsular opacification (PCO). PCO occurs in 100% of the patients at some point after cataract surgery, but not all patients need treatment. During cataract surgery the lens contents are removed and the emptied capsular bag remains in place. Some lens epithelial cells will remain on the capsular bag after the surgery. These remaining lens epithelial cells transform into fibroblast-like cells. They migrate over the surface of the capsular bag, produce extracellular matrix material and cause contraction of the capsular bag, leading to wrinkles. As a result, the optical axis can become opacified again, leading to visual complaints by the patient. PCO is usually treated by capsulotomy with an Nd-YAG laser. With this laser, a photodisruption of the central posterior capsule is created, resulting in a central hole. This allows for visual rehabilitation in most cases, but serious complications may also result. These include damage to or subluxation of the intraocular lens, retinal breaks, or retinal detachment.

Recently it was discovered that intraocular lenses with sharp edges to their optics exhibit significantly less PCO requiring treatment with the Nd-Yag laser. This has been attributed to a barrier effect of the sharp lens optic edge. Proliferating lens epithelial cells do not seem to be capable of passing the junction of the lens capsule with the sharp optic edge and this prevents proliferation of the lens epithelial cells towards the center of the lens capsule, keeping the lens capsule clear in the center. As a result of this, the rate of clinically significant PCO requiring Nd-Yag laser treatment is 5% three years after implantation of the intraocular lens. Before the discovery of the sharp-edge effect, Nd-Yag laser treatment was necessary in up to 30% of cases. In conclusion, PCO will occur in most patients, but due to the barrier effect of the edge of the lens optic, treatment will not be necessary in most patients.

> Posterior capsular opacification occurs after every cataract surgery.

Another complication of cataract surgery is rupture of the lens capsule during surgery. This occurs in 2–3% of all cataract procedures. The amount of damage to the lens capsule may vary. If the capsular bag can no longer support a posterior chamber lens, then another method of lens fixation has to be used (for instance, iris fixation). Rupture of the lens capsule may also disturb the vitreous body, which is behind the posterior lens capsule. Such disturbances may cause traction on the vitreous, leading to retinal breaks and retinal detachment. After rupture of the posterior capsule, all prolapsing vitreous has to be removed carefully, because it may compromise proper placement of the intraocular lens. The occurrence of a rupture of the capsular bag may have no negative side effects on the outcome of the cataract surgery when it is well treated, but the chance for vision-threatening complications is increased.

A third, potentially devastating complication after cataract surgery is endophthalmitis. In this condition, bacteria from the conjunctival flora cause a severe inflammation in the eye. This infection usually manifests itself within the first week after cataract surgery and the condition of the eye can deteriorate very rapidly. Within hours, a patient with good vision may become almost blind. When it is treated very rapidly, the eye and some vision may be saved, but in most patients the outcome is poor. Treatment consists of removal of a small sample of the vitreous body for culture and injection of antibiotics and anti-inflammatory drugs in the eye. A vitrectomy, removal of most of the vitreous body, may also be necessary to remove opacifications and inflammatory debris. Endophthalmitis occurs in approximately 0.1% of cataract procedures. Among risk factors for endophthalmitis are prolonged, complicated surgery and an immune-compromised patient (for instance due to diabetes mellitus).

> Endophthalmitis is a devastating complication of intraocular surgery.

It has been shown that preoperative application of povidon-iodine drops to the conjunctiva helps to decrease the incidence of endophthalmitis.[8] Furthermore, adherence to all usual rules for asepsis in the surgical theatre is necessary. In order to minimize the possibility of introducing bacteria in the eye via the intraocular lens, surgeons use injector systems to implant foldable intraocular lenses in the eye (see Fig. 5). This method of implantation reduces the number of contacts between possibly contaminated surgical instruments and the lens.

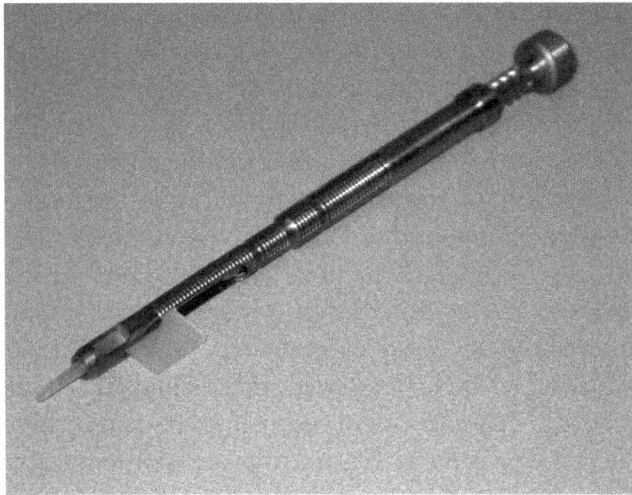

Fig. 5. Injector for intraocular lenses. By rotating the posterior end of the instrument, the plunger is advanced and the intraocular lens is pushed through the plastic cartridge where it folds and is delivered into the eye.

Intraocular lenses are implanted with forceps or with injection systems.

New Developments in Intraocular Lenses

Although intraocular lens implantation is very successful and leads to the restoration of sight in most patients, scientists are still looking for ways to improve lenses. By improving the implant lens optics, it is hoped that contrast vision of patients may be improved.[9] Effort is also being put toward trying to make intraocular lenses that can be implanted through the smaller incisions.

Another item to which much attention is given is the possibility to develop an intraocular lens which offers accommodation. Pseudophakic people usually need reading glasses after cataract surgery. An accommodative intraocular lens could correct presbyopia and allow patients to see clearly at all distances without glasses.[10]

Biomaterials Used in Posterior Segment Surgery

Most serious problems in the posterior segment of the eye that require surgery are caused by problems with the vitreous. The vitreous is the clear jelly-like substance that fills the central cavity of the eye, and is attached to the retina. It is most strongly attached to the retina at the periphery, but is also attached to the optic nerve.

As a person ages, the vitreous liquefies. With movements of the eye, the liquefied vitreous moves around inside the vitreous cavity. With time, the vitreous can pull free and separate from the retina and optic nerve. This is called posterior vitreous detachment and is a normal aging process. Because of the strong attachments of the vitreous to the retina in the periphery (the vitreous base), tugging can cause tears in the retina. The aging vitreous body may cause tears in the retina, leading to retinal detachment. If a tear occurs, it is a potentially serious problem. Fluid vitreous can pass through the tear and get under the retina, thereby causing a retinal detachment (see Fig. 6). Vision is lost wherever the retina becomes detached.

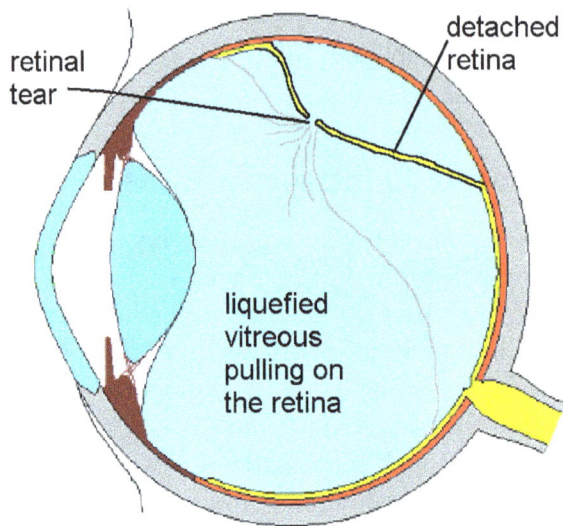

Fig. 6.   Posterior vitreous detachment causing a retinal tear and retinal detachment.

Without treatment vision is usually lost due to total retinal detachment. The incidence of retinal detachment is approximately one out of every 10,000 people. Certain people have a greater chance than others: people with high nearsightedness, a family history of retinal detachment, and patients who have had cataract surgery.

The traditional surgery for retinal detachment is scleral buckling surgery, which involves the use of encircling bands and explants to indent and compress the retina from the outside. The aim of surgery is closure of the retinal tear. This is accomplished by first treating the retinal tear with cryotherapy. A cryoprobe is placed on the outside of the eye in the correct position to treat the tear. Then a piece of silicone plastic is sewn onto the outside wall of the eye over the site of the tear (see Fig. 7). This pushes the sclera towards the retinal tear and holds the retina against the sclera until scarring from the cryotherapy seals the tear. The silicone buckle is left in place permanently. This is usually well tolerated by the eye.

In the 1980s a new hydrogel (Miragel©) buckle was marketed. This new buckle material seemed well tolerated and less prone to infection

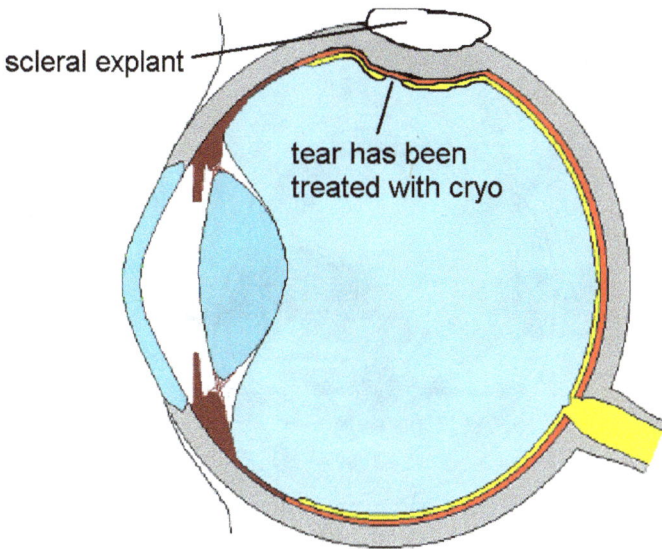

scleral explant

tear has been
treated with cryo

Fig. 7. Treatment of retinal detachment by a scleral buckle and cryotherapy.

due to its microporous surface. After a few years of worldwide use the first reports surfaced about swelling and degradation of the hydrogel causing different complications. Miragel was taken off the market.

For more complex retinal detachments, removal of the vitreous is necessary. This is called vitrectomy (see Fig. 8). Instruments are passed through 1 mm incisions in the sclera. The surgeon uses a fiber optic to illuminate the inside of the eye. With other instruments in the eye, such as a vitreous aspirator and cutter, forceps or scissors, vitreous, strands and fibrotic scars can be removed. Air, a gas mixture or a clear viscous fluid, silicone oil, replaces the vitreous. A gas mixture is absorbed over time by the eye and replaced by the eye's own fluid. The eye does not replace the vitreous itself. The lack of vitreous does not affect the functioning of the eye.

> Complex retinal detachments require removal and replacement of the vitreous body by a biomaterial.

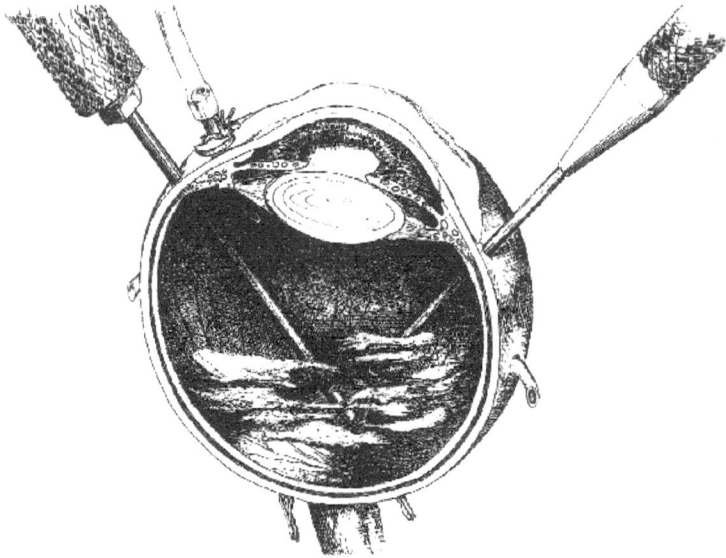

Fig. 8.   Treatment of vitreous and retinal pathology by vitrectomy.

For the most complex retinal detachments a long-term tampon-ade of the retina is necessary. The most widely used agent is silicone oil, a clear viscous fluid consisting of polydimethylsiloxanes with various chain length and molecular weight. Although most vitreo-retinal surgeons use silicone oil, it is far from the ideal tamponading agent.

The ideal vitreous substitute should be transparent, have long-term biocompatibility, have a high water-/tamponade-interface sur-face tension, low specific gravity for tamponade of superior retinal breaks and a high specific gravity for tamponade of inferior retinal breaks, a low viscosity for ease of handling, a low disperivity, and conformity to irregular surfaces.

Biomaterials have and will continue to have a vital place in eye surgery. Biomaterials used on the outside of the eye are satisfactory as surgical failure is rarely caused by materials complications. In contrast, vitreous substitutes are still far from ideal. The search for better substitutes is on.

References

1. Le Grand Y, El Hage SG. (1980) *Physiological Optics*. Springer-Verlag, Berlin, p. 29.
2. Dubbelman M van der, Heijde GL. (2001) The shape of the aging human lens: curvature, equivalent refractive index and the lens paradox. *Vision Research* 41:1867–77.
3. Thylefors B, Negrel AD, Pararajasegaram R, Dadzie KY. (1995) Global data on blindness. *Bull World Health Org* 73:115–21.
4. Congdon NG, Taylor HR. (2003) Age-related cataract. In: Johnson GJ, Minassian DC *et al.* (eds.), *The Epidemiology of Eye Disease*. Arnold, London, p. 105.
5. Kwitko ML, Kelman CD (eds.) (1998) *The History of Modern Cataract Surgery*. Kugler publications, The Hague.
6. Laeven AMW, Huijsmans H *et al.* (2000) *De achterkant van de wachtlijst*. Prismant, Utrecht, p. 44.
7. Apple DJ. (2003) A pioneer in the quest to eradicate world blindness. *Bulletin of the World Health Organization* 81:756–7.
8. Speaker MG, Menikoff JA. (1991) Prophylaxis of endophthalmitis with topical povidone-iodine. *Ophthalmology* 98(12):1769–75.
9. Packer M, Fine IH, Hoffman RS, Piers PA. (2002) Prospective randomized trial of an anterior surface modified prolate intraocular lens. *J Refract Surg* 18(6):692–6.
10. Waring GO III. (1992) Presbyopia and accommodative intraocular lenses — the next frontier in refractive surgery? *Refract Corneal Surg* 8(6):421–3.
11. Apple DJ, Ram J, Foster A, Peng Q. (2000) Elimination of cataract blindness. A global perspective entering the new millennium. *Surv Ophthalmol* 46(Suppl):1–196.

Case 6

Biomaterials in
Plastic Surgery

M.F. Meek*

Plastic surgery is a very broad surgical specialism covering recon-structive, aesthetic, craniofacial, congenital, burn, and hand sur-gery. This implies that plastic surgeons operate on a diverse patient population and almost all anatomical sites of the body, both sexes, and all ages.

There are many applications of biomaterials in plastic surgery. One can think of joint reconstruction, osteosynthesis (e.g. plates and screws), reconstruction and creation of the shapes of bones and soft tissues (e.g. breast reconstruction and augmentation), glues, suture materials, and injectables.

Introduction

Polymeric biomaterials that are generally regarded as safe now may not be considered safe in the future. The surgeon who implants a biomaterial may have to deal with a malpractice situation many years

*Plastic, Hand and Peripheral Nerve Surgeon, Pulvertaft Hand Centre, Derbyshire Royal Infirmary, London Road, Derby DE1 2QY, U.K.

after the implant was placed. This is exactly the situation now faced by some plastic surgeons.

If autologous tissue is available and will adequately solve the problem, it should be used preferentially. If autologous material is not available or will result in obvious donor morbidity, or not solve the problem, the surgeon should select only those implants with the lowest potential for future problems.

FDA and CE approvals are of importance in order to know that the biomaterial is biocompatible, and resorbs without any disadvantages (in case of resorbable products), especially for clinicians who have relatively little experience or biomaterial knowledge.

The use of biomaterials has become an essential part in reconstructive and aesthetic procedures in plastic surgery. This chapter provides a brief introduction and case studies in order to give more insight into some of the commonly used implant materials available in this profession.

Metacarpophalangeal Joint Reconstruction in a Rheumatoid Arthritis Patient

Rheumatoid arthritis is a systemic autoimmune disease which is characterized by an inflammatory synovial response as its predominant feature, with bone and cartilage destruction being secondary to this.

The main aims of joint reconstruction are alleviation of pain and improvement of the normal anatomy (position) and range of motion of the joint. The metacarpophalangeal joint is the most commonly involved joint when rheumatoid arthritis affects the hand (see Fig. 1). Many prosthetic implants have been designed for the replacement of this joint, and Swanson silicone implants have long been the "gold standard" of metacarpophalangeal joint reconstruction in rheumatoid arthritis patients (see Fig. 2). However, durability problems (e.g. implant failure and particulate synovitis) of silicone implants have led to the use of other implants as well.

Anatomy

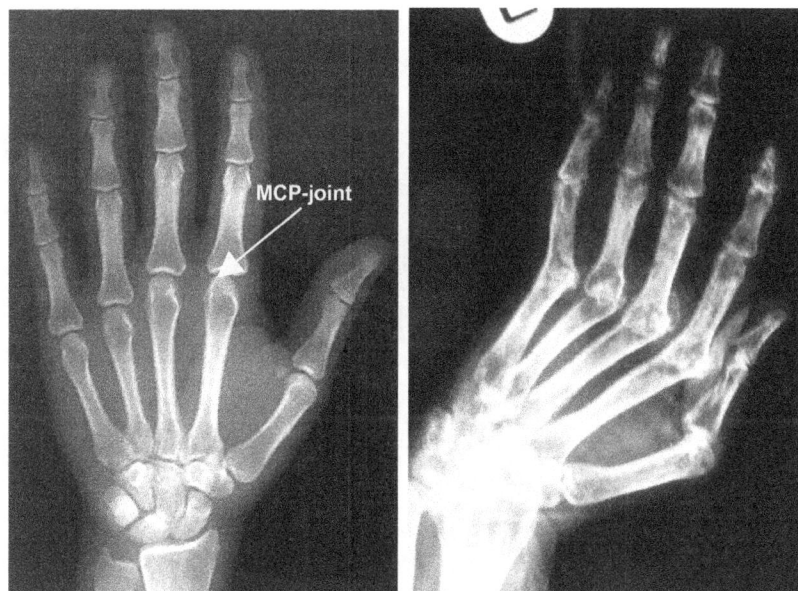

Fig. 1. X-ray of a hand with normal anatomy (left). X-ray of a rheumatoid hand (right).

Peripheral Nerve Reconstruction

A peripheral nerve carries information to and from the brain and spinal cord to the outer frontiers of the body and connects with peripheral receptors or effectors. Motor nerves carry messages from the brain to muscles to make the body move, while sensory nerves carry messages to the brain from different parts of the body to signal pain, pressure and temperature. The axon nerve fiber carries only one type of message, either motor or sensory; most nerves in the body are made up of both.

After a peripheral nerve is injured with loss of continuity, the nerve is not able to carry information anymore (see Figs. 3A and B). Only the part connected to the central nervous system survives. To re-obtain nerve function, nerve continuity has to be re-established.

Application

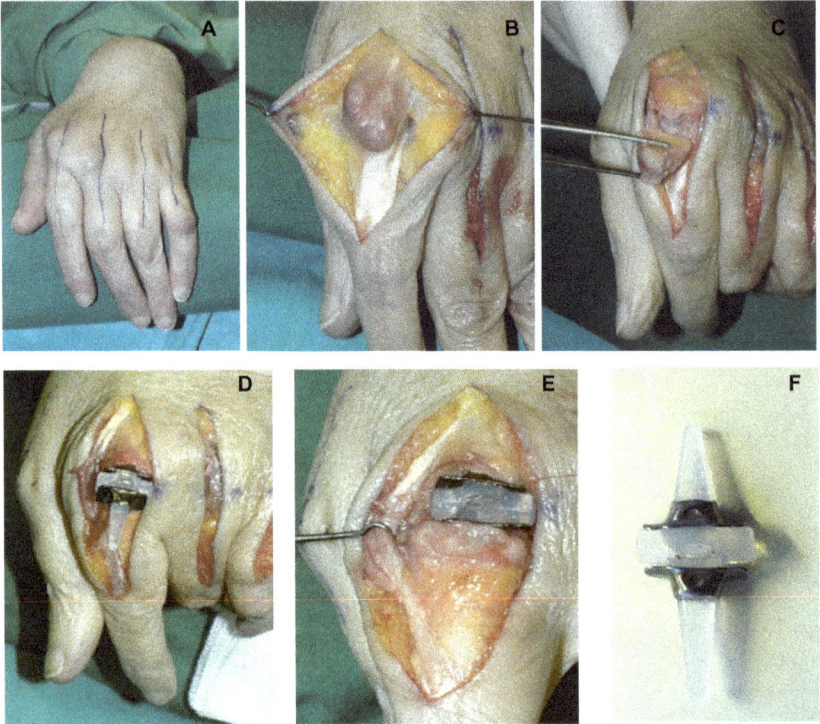

Fig. 2.   (**A**) preoperative drawings on a rheumatoid hand; (**B**) a rheumatoid nodule is visible; (**C**) the rheumatoid nodule is excised and the proximal part of the MCP joint is excised; (**D**) MCP joint prosthetic implant in the second metacarpal after reaming; (**E**) MCP joint prosthetic implant in the second metacarpal and the proximal phalanx of the index finger; (**F**) MCP joint prosthetic implant.

The standard technique for bridging a peripheral nerve defect is an autologous nerve graft, if the nerve ends cannot be sutured. Recently, research was performed into a possible alternative: a biodegradable nerve guide (see Fig. 3C).

A 28-year-old man cut his left non-dominant thumb accidentally with a piece of glass. He had normal sensation at the radial side of the tip of the thumb, whereas sensation was absent at the ulnar side. In Fig. 4 a schematic representation can be seen of the normal peripheral nerve innervation of the thumb and a defect in the ulnar

Anatomy

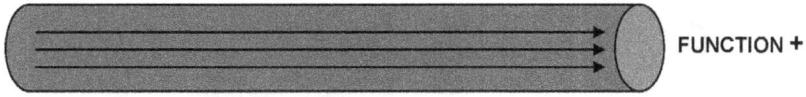

A. Intact peripheral nerve with normal nerve conduction (arrows), normal nerve function.

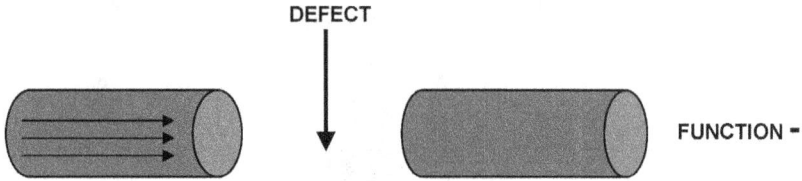

B. Peripheral nerve defect; no nerve conduction over the defect, no nerve function.

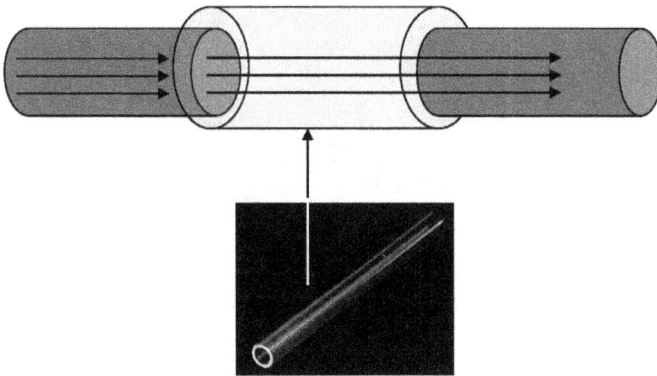

C. Bridging the nerve defect with a nerve guide in order to regain nerve function

Fig. 3.   Figure shows the use of a nerve guide for repair of a peripheral nerve defect.

digital nerve of the thumb (see Fig. 4B). A biodegradable nerve guide was used to bridge the defect of approximately 5 mm (see Fig. 5).

Injectable Synthetic Soft Tissue Fillers

Several soft tissue fillers are available, with more than 100 different fillers used worldwide. They can be distinguished into synthetic fillers, biological fillers, homologous fillers and autologous fillers. This

Application

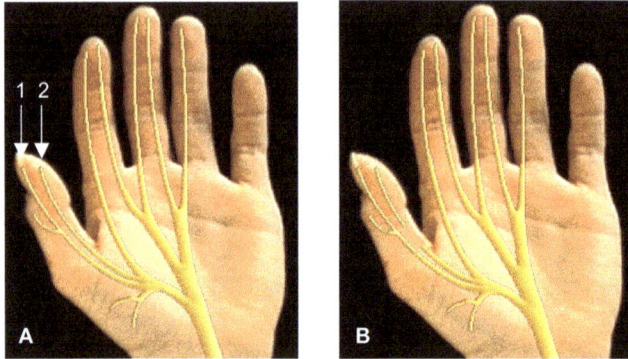

Fig. 4. (**A**) 1. Radial digital nerve of the thumb. 2. Ulnar digital nerve of the thumb.
(**B**) Defect in the ulnar digital nerve of the thumb.

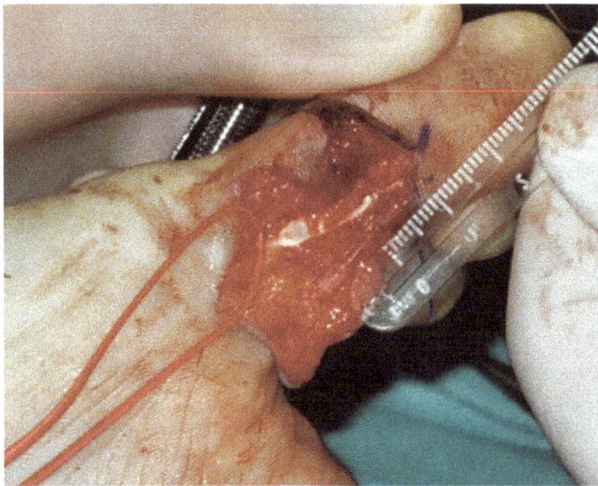

Fig. 5. Biodegradable nerve guide used for the repair of a gap of approximately
5 mm in the ulnar digital nerve of the thumb.

chapter is focused upon synthetic fillers, which can be used to create
permanent soft tissue augmentation.

There are several synthetic fillers available. Silicone oil, for example, can be injected in microdroplets into the subdermis (see also

Anatomy

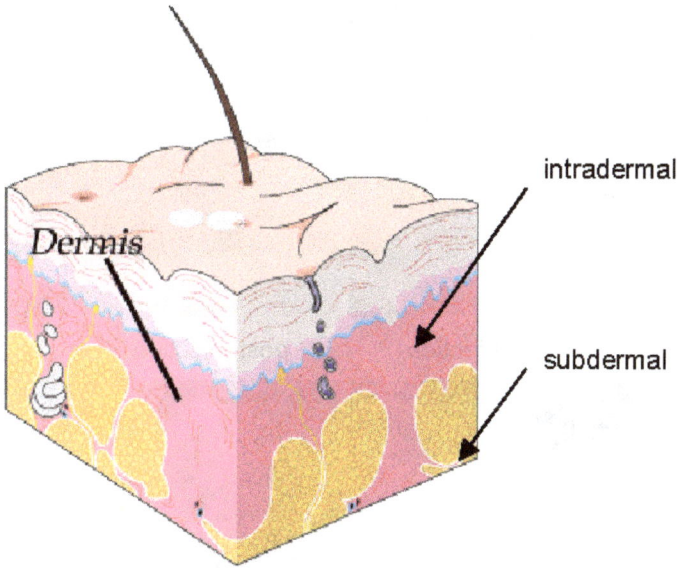

Fig. 6.   Cross section of the skin. Some injectables are injected into the dermis, others are injected subdermally.

Fig. 6). A fibrous capsule will be formed around each capsule, resulting in augmentation. However, silicone is difficult to remove once it is injected. Another example of a synthetic filler is solid silicone particles suspended in a polyvinylpyrridolone $(C_6H_9NO)_n$ carrier (Bioplastique). It can be injected subcutaneously. Before the injectable is placed, the area is infiltrated with lidocaine and epinephrine for anesthesia and vasoconstriction.

Microspheres of polymethylmethacrylate (PMMA) suspended in a gelatin/bovine collagen solution (Arteplast and Artecoll) are also used as synthetic fillers. The solution degrades in 1–3 months, and the microspheres will be encapsulated within 2–4 months. PMMA is injected into the subdermis.

The indications for fillers are soft tissue augmentation for correction of post-surgical or post-traumatic defects, certain diseases (e.g. lipodystrofia in HIV patients), correction of folds and wrinkles, and lip enhancement (see Fig. 7).

Application

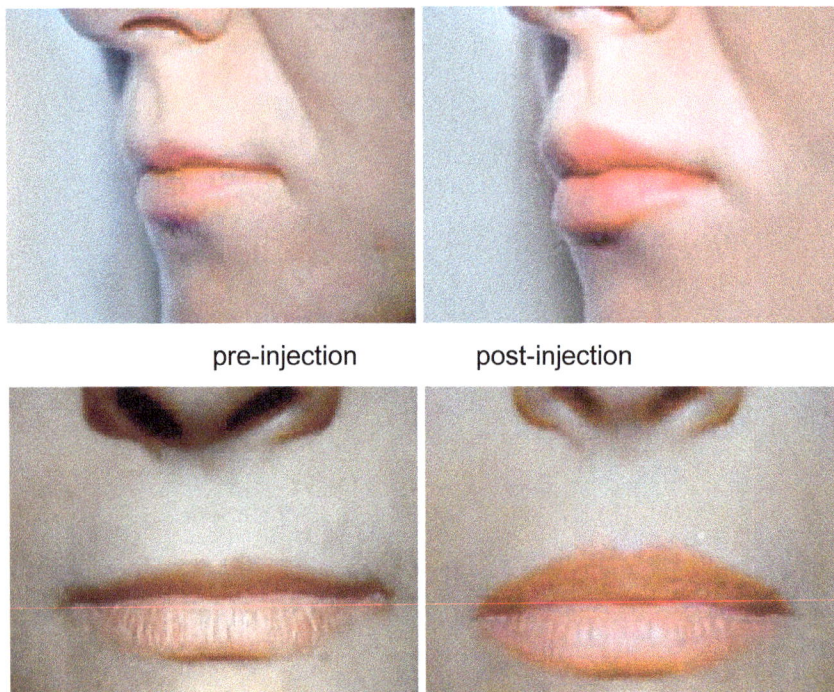

pre-injection   post-injection

Fig. 7.   Example of a cosmetic augmentation of the lips by injection.

Complications arising from the use of synthetic materials will probably increase in number because of the increasing number of injectables that are becoming available. Non-resorbable fillers can lead to permanent damage. Complications can occur because of the body's reaction to the product, incorrect utilization, or composition of the product. Many complications have been described with the use of synthetic fillers: inflammation, granulomas, edema, erythema, nodules at the injection site, pain, abscess formation, induration, dislocation, ulceration, migration, pruritis, hypertrophic scarring, and allergic reaction. In some countries (e.g. Switzerland) non-resorbable products are discouraged by the authorities for purely esthetic indications.

The ideal injectable soft tissue filler has not yet been identified. It should offer reproducible results, be easy to use, be safe (e.g. biocompatible, nonpyrogenic, nontoxic, noncarcinogenic, nonallergenic, nonimmunogenic), and with minimal complications and risk of migration. At the moment there is a lack of prospective randomized trials in this field.

The person that injects soft tissue filler should have a thorough knowledge of the available options and their risks. Very often injectables are used by people who have no medical background. The author of this chapter, however, believes that the person who injects filler into a patient/client should not only be able to inject, but also solve any possible complications arising from the injection. Sometimes complications may occur at a later stage, necessitating the removal of the injectable by using a surgical reduction. These procedures should only be carried out by board-certified medical specialists capable of providing the patient with the highest care possible. A very good development is the rule in Switzerland that only medical doctors or nurses under their direct supervision are allowed to perform injections of products intended to stay in the patient for more than 30 days.

Breast Augmentation

Breast augmentation is a surgical procedure to enhance the size and shape of a breast. The reason for breast augmentation can be to correct the reduction of breast volume after pregnancy, to balance a difference in breast size, or as a reconstructive technique following breast surgery.

Several techniques are available for breast augmentation (see Fig. 8). The implants can be placed subglandularly, submuscularly or in dual plane. Subglandular placement offers a natural positioning and movement, and has the added benefit of quick recovery time with little post-surgical discomfort. It can also sometimes lift small or sagging breasts. Submuscular implants tend to work better for women who are very thin and therefore do not have very much

Anatomy

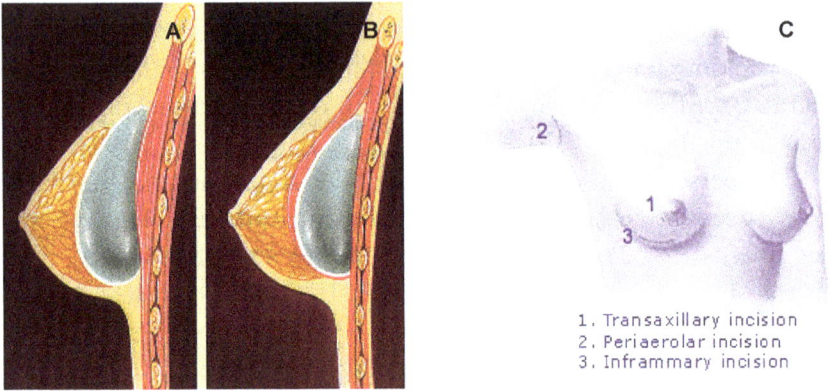

1. Transaxillary incision
2. Periaerolar incision
3. Inframmary incision

Fig. 8.   Examples of positioning of breast implants: subglandular (**A**), and submuscular (**B**). In C, several incisions through which the implants can be brought into the right place.

breast tissue to fully cover the implant. Submuscular placement can help to hide the implant and may reduce the possibility of rippling or capsular contracture (hardening of the breast). Submuscular placement also offers more fullness towards the top of the breasts. This technique requires slightly longer recovery time compared with subglandular implants. Dual plane placement places the implant partially above and partially below the muscle. In theory, this technique takes advantage of the subglandular and submuscular procedures, resulting in natural breasts with a full cleavage and low risk of rippling or capsular contracture. Breast implants may vary in shell surface (smooth versus textured), shape (round or shaped) (see Fig 9), profile (how far they stick out), volume (size), shell thickness, and filler material. There are several complications that may occur. Capsular contracture happens when the scar tissue or capsule that normally forms around the implant tightens and squeezes the implant. Rupture/deflation may occur, and breast implants rarely last a lifetime. Other possible complications include pain, and nipple and breast sensation changes. In Fig. 10, an example of breast augmentation can be seen.

Application

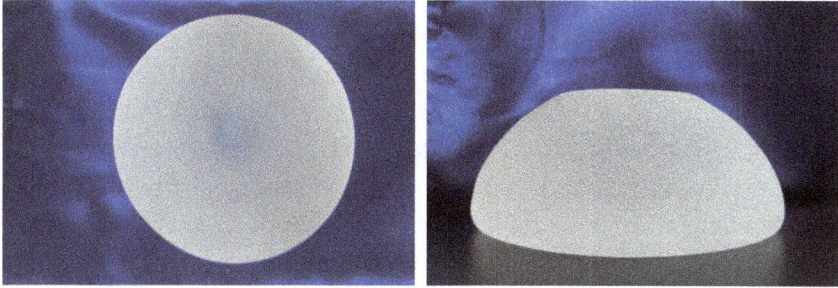

Fig. 9. Example of a round silicone gel-filled breast implant.

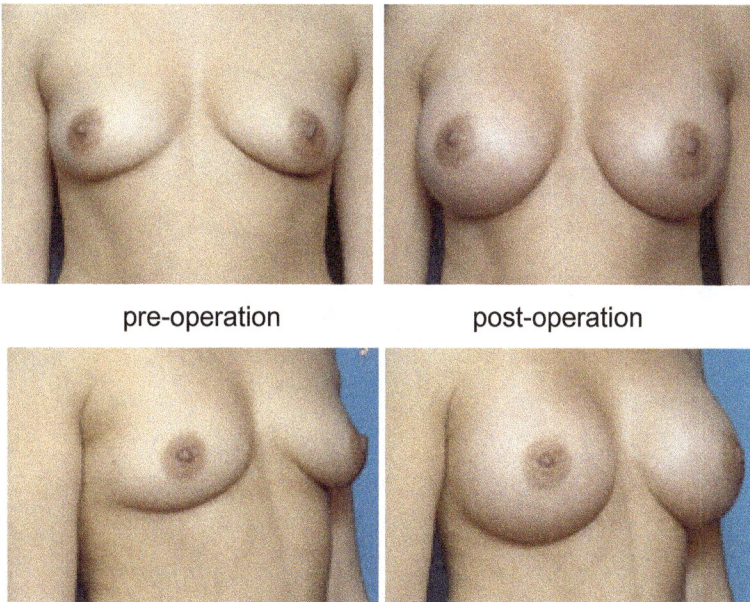

pre-operation　　　　post-operation

Fig. 10. Pre- and post-operative pictures of breast augmentation.

Closure

Following on the evolution of biomaterials, tissue engineering is now seeing the increased introduction of (degradable) scaffolds with growth factors. Combining biomedical engineering and polymer science together with clinical input and applications, mainly in surgical specialities, has led to several biomaterial applications in the clinic. A new field of research coming up is the use of stem cells in order to direct the outgrowth of several specific autologous tissue lines in order to repair or reconstruct tissue defects. It will take several years, but we can expect FDA- and CE-approved cell cultures and constructs in the near future. New biomedical applications launched in plastic surgery should always show extra value against the available products already on the market.

Case 7

Surgical Meshes — Morphology-dependent Bacterial Colonization

A.F. Engelsman*

Abdominal wall hernia repairs are the second most common surgical procedure performed in the USA, behind only cataract procedures. Although surgical techniques in hernia repair have improved, recurrence used to be a common complication. Therefore, the idea of increasing the strength of the abdominal wall by implanting a mesh was explored. The introduction of a polypropylene mesh in 1962 was a breakthrough with regards to biocompatibility and comfort. The positive effects of the use of a mesh on recurrence of the hernia stimulated the search for an optimal mesh with biocompatibility, low adhesion formation and low infection rates. To date a large number of surgical meshes are available for abdominal wall reconstruction. They all differ concerning tissue ingrowth, change of infection and rate of recurrence. The enormous variety in materials available implies important differences concerning interactions between surgical mesh and micro-organisms. To date, the use of a

*Department of BioMedical Engineering, University Medical Center Groningen, A. Deusinglaan 1, 9713 AV Groningen, The Netherlands.

surgical mesh always forces the clinician to choose between the risks of prosthesis-related complications and a suboptimal treatment without a device and high rates of recurrence.[a]

Clinical Background to Abdominal Wall Defects

An abdominal wall defect or abdominal hernia is defined as a protrusion through the abdominal wall of intra-abdominal content with an intact lining of the sac. Figure 1A illustrates the normal anatomical situation, with the peritoneum covering the entire abdominal cavity. Also, the relation between the main anatomical structures, such as the abdominal cavity, abdominal muscles and fasciae, aorta, and spine is shown. Figure 1B demonstrates a midline abdominal wall defect due to detachment of the bilateral rectus abdominis muscles. A hernia sac lined with peritoneum protrudes (arrow) through the hernial port of the abdominal fascia and muscles and is bilaterally enclosed by the rectus abdominis muscle. A protrusion can occur when the abdominal wall is exposed to chronically elevated intra-abdominal pressure, e.g. due to prostatism, constipation, high physical workload or chronic cough in patients with obstructive pulmonary disease. In this group of patients, hernia repairs can be successful; however, surgical treatment should be accompanied with sufficient post-operative advice to the patient and appropriate lowering of the intra-abdominal pressure. Patient activity and technical factors are held responsible for early recurrences after hernia repair. Late recurrences are mainly related to aging factors or affected collagen build-up.

The integrity of the abdominal wall is important for both the physical and physiological well-being of the patient. Defects enhance malfunction of musculature and the stability of position and balance of the human body. Most hernias are diagnosed upon physical examination as a bulge at the site of the hernia increasing with coughing or straining. Abdominal wall defects can be accompanied by a spectrum of symptoms, including profound peritoneal signs when

---

[a] Parts are published in: Engelsman AF, *et al.* (2007) The phenomenon of infection with abdominal wall reconstruction. *Biomaterials* 28:2314–27.

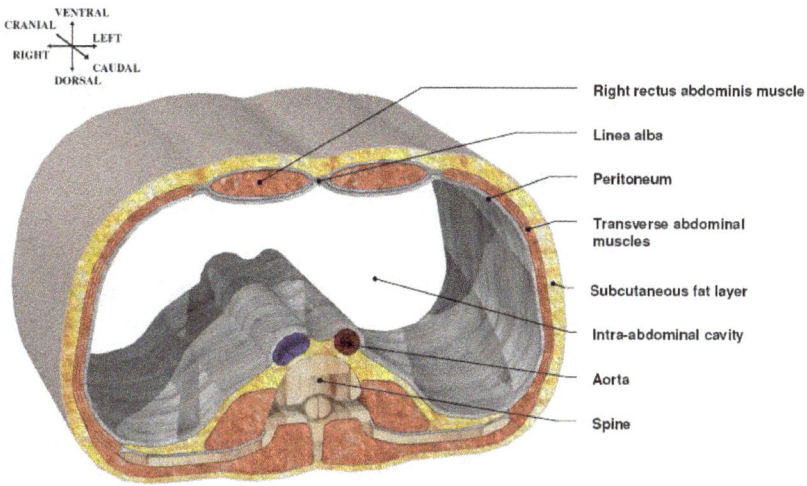

Fig. 1A. A schematic presentation of the normal anatomy of the abdominal wall.

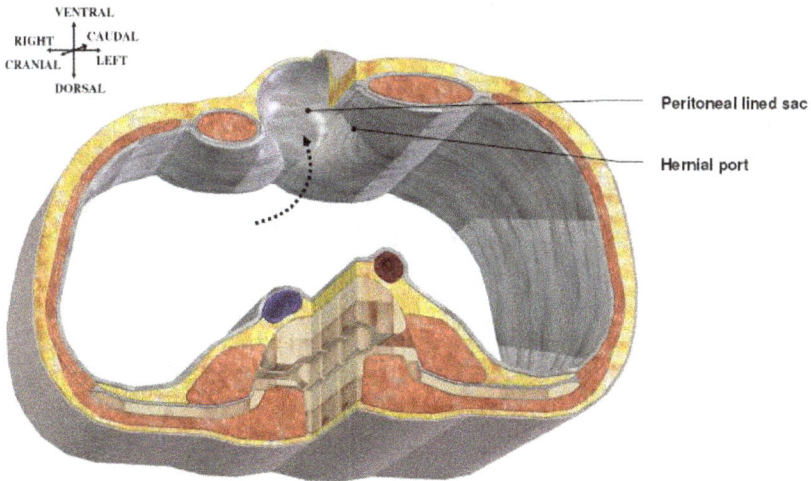

Fig. 1B. The mechanism of an abdominal wall defect.

strangulation of intra-abdominal structures occurs. The most common symptom is a heavy or dull sense of discomfort during straining or lifting. Strangulation of abdominal contents in the hernial port is a major complication of any abdominal wall defect and is most common in small and newly formed hernias. Strangulation of abdominal contents usually presents with extreme pain and an acute abdomen and may lead to acute small bowel obstruction due to tissue ischemia, necrosis, peritonitis and septicaemia requiring extensive resection of the intestine. All these factors can result in extensive morbidity for defects of the abdominal wall, which will result in social and financial losses.

The only effective treatment for abdominal wall defects is surgery to restore integrity and maintain function of the abdominal wall and prevent incarceration and strangulation of intra-abdominal content. In the past, hernia surgery and abdominal wall reconstructions have frequently used tense sutures to approximate and close a hernial port or defect. With this technique, wound dehiscence, recurrent hernias, and non-healing of the wound due to tissue ischemia, with the sutures cutting through the soft tissue, are frequent. The successful repair of an abdominal wall defect is based on a tension-free closure to allow wound repair, a better collagen restoration and prevention of recurrence. A tension-free closure may be accomplished by applying a technique following Ramirez *et al.*,[1] which replaces the need of a mesh, but requires extensive surgery, or by the placement of a surgical mesh to relieve tension from tissue surrounding the hernial port.

Surgical Meshes in Abdominal Wall Repairs

The use of tissue-supporting meshes allows a tension-free solution for the repair of abdominal wall defects, which has decreased the recurrence rates in hernia surgery dramatically. Due to the improved clinical outcome, the use of surgical meshes has steadily increased over the years. Worldwide, an estimated 1 million synthetic meshes are used annually in surgery. To allow the placement of the mesh between the external fascial layer and the rectus abdominis muscles, the abdominal wall has to be opened. After reducing the hernial sac into the abdominal cavity the defect is covered with a surgical mesh (see Fig. 1C). With the availability of meshes an intra-abdominal approach to repair an abdominal defect using laparoscopic techniques also became feasible. Laparoscopic abdominal wall reconstruction is minimally invasive, results in only small wounds, and yields lower recurrence and infection

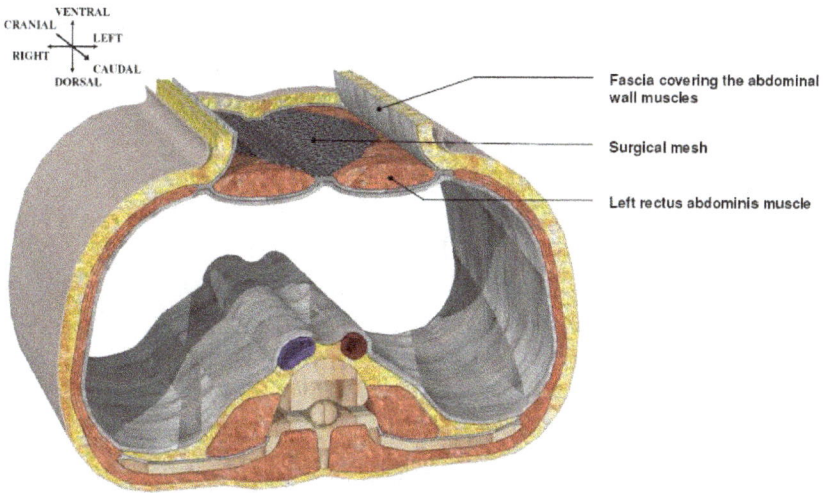

Fig. 1C. Through the "open technique," implantation of a surgical mesh.

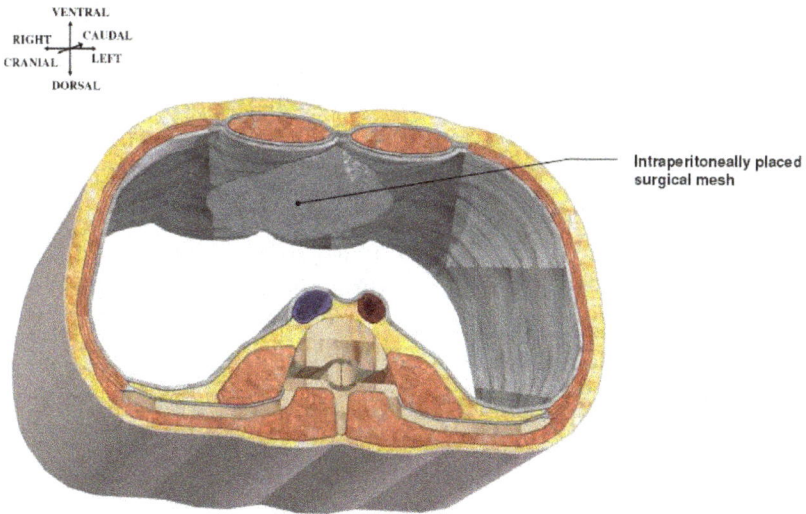

Fig. 1D. Intraperitoneal placement of a surgical mesh.

rates. Figure 1D illustrates the placement of an intra-abdominally placed mesh by means of laparoscopic surgery covering the internal hernial port. The most frequent complications following the use of mesh are intra-abdominal adhesions and erosion of the intestines.

The strength of the abdominal wall depends on the collagen fascia layers, which, in fact, are the structures to be replaced by a proper mesh. From a mechanical point of view, abdominal wall implants should become an integrated part of the abdominal wall. This requires complete incorporation of the mesh into the fascial margins of the defect. In the repair of abdominal wall defects, surgical meshes can either be placed fully intra-abdominally (on the surface of the peritoneal lining) or in between different anatomical layers of the abdominal wall. In both situations the aim of the treatment is to consolidate a musculo-fascial defect without tension on the surrounding tissues.

Since the introduction of polypropylene (PP) in the 1960s in abdominal wall reconstructive surgery, two more polymers have been used to construct non-absorbable synthetic meshes: polyester (POL), and polytetrafluorethylene (PTFE). PP is highly biocompatible, which results in easy host tissue ingrowth, and thus the formation of adhesions. Therefore, its application is contraindicated when the mesh may be in direct contact with the intestines (see Fig. 1D), but is of great use when placed in between the fascial layers (see Fig. 1C). Severe adhesion formation with PP and POL meshes causing bowel obstruction, subsequent erosion and the formation of fistulas when placed in direct contact with the intestine have been reported. In contrast, ePTFE, with its low tissue ingrowth rates due to its hydrophobic nature, does not show these effects and, therefore, is preferred for intra-abdominal use.

The amount of material used as surgical mesh affects the extent of the reaction of host tissue and directly influences the amount of collagen deposition. A lightweight mesh is constructed with a small amount of material and large pores (e.g. Lars®), in contrast to a heavyweight mesh (e.g. Bard Teflon® mesh). A heavyweight non-absorbable mesh induces a much stronger host tissue reaction compared to lightweight meshes or absorbable meshes, which results in a thicker collagen plate and, ultimately, more patient discomfort. Due to their better abdominal wall compliance and the lower levels of chronic pain caused, lightweight meshes are favored for implantation in the abdominal wall compared to heavyweight meshes. A balance between the host tissue response and the mesh material should be sought in the development of surgical meshes.

Despite its advantages, the use of a biomaterial in abdominal wall reconstructive surgery also increases the risk of complications, such as mesh-related infection, intestinal adhesion formation and general discomfort. An infected implant becomes especially trouble-some when a biofilm is formed. Micro-organisms in this biofilm are armed against the host's immune response and antimicrobial meas-ures. This will often lead to major complications, which can be potentially life-threatening, and will in the majority of cases result in removal of the mesh. Despite these concerns, the use of a mesh remains superior to a suture repair with regard to recurrence rates, regardless of the size and location of the hernia.

Classification of Surgical Meshes

Significant differences exist between the available surgical meshes. These differences include type of material, amount of yarns and type of construction (see also Table 1 for a brief overview). These differ-ences influence ingrowth of host tissue, as well as bacterial attach-ment and growth on the implant. Meshes can be classified based on their weight per square meter. In this case, lightweight and heavy-weight meshes are distinguished, but a consensus for these defini-tions is not available. Amid *et al.* classified surgical meshes based on their pore size, distinguishing four groups: group I with pores larger than 75 μm; group II with pores smaller than 75 μm; group III with a macro-porous structure, but containing micro-porous aspects; and group IV incorporating all organic materials. This chapter distin-guishes absorbable synthetic, non-absorbable synthetic and organic materials.

Non-Absorbable Synthetic Materials

Synthetic materials are made of polymer chains which offer the bene-fit of off-the-shelf availability when they are needed. For a synthetic material to be accepted for clinical use, it has to be incorporated

Table 1. Scanning Electron Images of Commonly Used Non-absorbable Surgical Meshes, Together with the Main Differences in Material Type, Wettability, Yarn Structure, Mesh Strength and Surface Area

Physical Appearance (SEM Picture)[2-4]	Trade Name	Material	Classi-fication[5]	Mesh Wettability (Degrees) (Front/Back)[3]	Number of Filaments	Yarn Ø $(\mu m)^{3,6}$	Filament Ø $(\mu m)^{3,6}$
	Marlex®	PP	I	122 ± 3 130 ± 6	Mono	161.6 ± 8.7	—
	Prolene®	PP	I	N.D.	Dual	153.1 ± 9.3	—
	Surgipro™	PP	III	N.D.	Multi	≈ 173	15.8 ± 1.6
N.A.	Trelex®	PP	I	116 ± 5 134 ± 3	Mono	185.9 ± 18.0	—
N.A.	Lars®	POL	III	N.D.	Multi	≈ 261	(16.8 ± 1.6) × (6.0 ± 1.0)
	Fluoro-passiv®	POL	III	68 ± 10	Multi	—	12.6 ± 1.4
	Gore-Tex®	ePTFE	II	111 ± 4	—	—	—
	Bard® Teflon	PTFE	III	99 ± 3	Multi	± 313	(22.3 ± 3.2) × (12.0 ± 2.9)

PP	polypropylene	CH3-[CH2-CH(CH3)]n-CH3
POL	polyester	HO-R-O-[CO-(CH2)4-CO-O-R-O]n-H
ePTFE	expanded polytetrafluorethylene	-[CF2-CF2]-
PTFE	polytetrafluorethylene	-[CF2-CF2]-
PG	polyglactin	
PLA	polyglycolic acid	-[O-CH(CH3)-CO-O]n-
N.D.	Not Determined	
N.A.	Not Available	

without extensive host tissue reaction, which implies a favorable interaction between host and implanted material. Since the introduction of polypropylene in 1962, four main groups of different materials have become available for abdominal wall reconstruction: PP, PTFE, expanded PTFE and POL. PP, POL and PTFE can be worked up in different ways (monofilament or multifilament yarns and with a knitted or woven structure) to form a broad variety of available meshes.

Table 1 lists a number of different meshes, including some mesh-specific features that influence collagen build-up and/or bacterial colonization. The yarn diameter and high tex-index (g/1000 m of yarn) of Bard Teflon® clearly show that this is a heavyweight mesh, which will induce a massive host tissue reaction. High water contact angles on the mesh means a hydrophobic surface (as seen with Marlex®, Gore-Tex® and Bard Teflon® meshes), which reduces the bacterial colonization of the meshes. In contrast, Fluoropassiv® mesh is more hydrophilic, as shown by the lower water contact angles, which is induced by a gelatin coating. A hydrophilic mesh promotes better biocompatibility during the first weeks after implantation. The advances of multifilament yarns are mainly practical, since a multifilament yarn increases its ease of use due to its increased flexibility. But, multifilament yarns are suggested to increase the opportunity for micro-organisms to attach to and colonize the mesh, due to a relative protection from the niches present in multifilament yarns.

Despite numerous new developments, monofilament PP remains the most commonly used material for surgical meshes. Its large pore size and biocompatibility allow relatively easy tissue ingrowth and inflammatory cell response on the surface of the material. However, there are growing problems concerning the use of PP mesh in the repair of large ventral hernias, as the meshes tend to shrink and migrate to neighboring organs while inducing the formation of dense adhesions with the intestines and even fistulization to the intestinal lumen. Formation of adhesions are a growing concern since the laparoscopic hernia repair technique, in which the mesh is placed in direct contact with the intestines, has proved successful in reducing infection rates and recurrence rates compared to open techniques. Therefore, with advanced laparoscopic techniques using intra-peritoneal placement of the mesh, new materials and modifications are being developed to cope with extensive adhesion formation. One example of a low-adhesive mesh is the Gore-Tex® Soft Tissue Patch. The micro-porous character of this material reduces the host tissue ingrowth rate, and thus the formation of adhesions, allowing ePTFE to be safely placed in direct contact with the intestines. At the same time, this aspect of ePTFE mesh reduces the accessibility of micro-organisms which are hidden in the porous material for the host immune system. Therefore, when ePTFE meshes are infected, treatment requires the removal of the device.

Absorbable Synthetic Materials

Absorbable materials for surgical meshes in reconstructive abdominal wall surgery have been developed because of the reported long-term risk of infection and patient morbidity when permanent, non- absorbable materials are used. Absorbable synthetic meshes contain glycolic acid (GA) and poly(lactic acid) compounds in different ratios. As far as degradation kinetics is concerned, it is known that degradation of absorbable meshes increases with increasing GA content. The most commonly used short-term absorbable meshes consist of polyglactin (PG) 910, a combination of glycolic and lactic acids in a ratio of 9:1. This material loses 50% of its tensile strength within 2–3 weeks, although, fragments of the polymer are detectable up to three months after implantation. In contrast, materials consisting of a combination of 95% lactic acid and 5% glycolic acid maintain their tensile strength for at least nine months. Theoretically, absorbable meshes give acute support in the defective abdominal wall and allow fibro-connective tissue to take over the functional repair when the mesh is completely absorbed. Nevertheless, studies with a long-term follow-up on absorbable materials have not provided any conclusive advantages as regards recurrence compared to suture repairs.

The massive formation of fibro-connective tissue around regular non-absorbable meshes is held responsible for patient complaints concerning restriction in mobility of the abdominal wall. The need for reduction of mesh material while retaining the required strength has resulted in composite meshes, in which absorbable and non-absorbable materials are combined. The combination of absorbable and non-absorbable materials gives acute strength during the first weeks after implantation. When the absorbable residue of the mesh is replaced by collagen fibers only a lightweight non-absorbable part ensures permanent strength in combination with low patient morbidity. Reduction of the mesh material by replacing non-absorbable material with absorbable material gives a combination of acute strength, long-term stability and a more flexible fibro-connective abdominal plate. Therefore, the future for the use of absorbable materials in abdominal wall reconstructive surgery lies in composite mesh grafts.

Organic Materials

Further development of organic meshes for abdominal wall reconstruction has mainly been stimulated by the persistence of complications with synthetic materials. Research and development in the field of organic materials for abdominal reconstruction is increasing, although organic materials do carry a number of additional risk factors compared with synthetic meshes (such as immunologic rejection and potential transmission of viral diseases). These materials, however, yield low bacterial infection rates and high biocompatibility; Ansaloni and colleagues compared the use of porcine small-intestinal submucosa (Surgisis®) to PP mesh and observed that post-hernioplasty acute and chronic discomfort and analgesic consumption were lower in the Surgisis® group.[7] Also, infection rates in a group of immunodeficient subjects, i.e. HIV-positive and transplant patients, were lower with the use of Surgisis®.

Mesh Infection

Infection is one of the most devastating complications that can follow implantation of any implant material, and is especially troublesome when a biofilm is formed on the mesh. Infection of a mesh results in increased patient morbidity due to secondary operations, impaired wound healing and functional loss of the abdominal wall, and significantly extended hospital stay. Primary abdominal wall reconstruction with a mesh is considered to be a clean surgery and the incidence of post-operative mesh infection is 1–2% of all grafts. Repairs of incisional hernias are considered to be contaminated surgery due to the significantly higher infection rates described with these repairs. Bacterial colonization of biomaterial surfaces will interfere with adequate host tissue integration.[8] Wound-infection is a risk-factor for recurrence of hernia, which stresses the need to prevent this situation in individual patients.

Bacterial colonization occurs in approximately one-third of all surgical meshes implanted, even after years of implantation, and also without clinical signs of infection. A large number of clinical studies have been published on infection rates of abdominal wall implants, demonstrating that the incidence of infection depends heavily on mesh type and the surgical technique applied. PP meshes show infection rates ranging from 2–4.2%. In contrast, ePTFE shows a broader range of infection rates, varying from 0–9.2% when an open surgical approach is used, and only 0–1% when a laparoscopic approach is used. Multifilament POL meshes show the highest infection percentages, ranging from 7–16%, while monofilament POL meshes show infection rates comparable with PP meshes. These clinical observations feed the assumption that multifilament yarns are more susceptible to bacterial colonization than monofilament yarns.

Scott *et al.*[9] reviewed 10 randomized prospective studies comparing open mesh with open non-mesh techniques for inguinal hernia repair. They showed significantly higher infection rates and a lower recurrence rate when mesh was used. Their results suggest that the incidence of recurrence is lowered with the introduction of mesh, but when infection occurs, problems concerning recurrence greatly increase. Infection that requires removal of the patch will generally result in recurrence, as this must be repaired primarily without the use of a mesh. On the other hand, the use of collagen mesh may allow immediate repair, but this is associated with a high failure rate. Therefore, a staged repair will be necessary in most patients.

The presence of micro-organisms has been demonstrated in zones of tissue repair and, specifically, in areas of chronic foreign body reactions. In the presence of a biomaterial, infection alters tissue infiltration and so interferes with the repair process, leading to significant changes in host tissue that may, in the abdominal wall, give rise to hernia recurrence and the need for replacement of the mesh. In several cases, removal of the infected biomaterial will be necessary to eradicate the infection, especially if the mesh contains a component of ePTFE.

Recently, a number of publications have described the onset of infection of the mesh involving abscess formation, with a significant delay of up to 39 months after implantation. A possible explanation for the delay of this complication is the continuing presence of bacteria from the introduction during surgery onward. In most cases the bacteria are protected from the immune response of the host and antibiotics by a biofilm and the presence of submicron niches and pores in the mesh structure.

Bacterial Properties Determining Colonization of an Implant Device

In order to adhere, bacteria undergo functional changes when they are in contact with a surface. Part of this process is the production of slime, which enhances an irreversible and strong adhesion. The metabolic changes that contribute to these functional alterations of attached micro-organisms have not been elucidated, but it has been suggested that this is almost solely induced by the surrounding environment. In general, slime-producing micro-organisms survive better on implant surfaces than non-slime producing micro-organisms and therefore, slime production is a major pathogenic property of bacterial strains that form biofilms on surfaces.

Staphylococcus epidermidis preferentially adheres to polymers, while *Staphylococcus aureus* prefers to adhere to metals, which explains why the former often causes polymer implant infection (e.g. catheters or meshes) and the latter is the major pathogen in metal implant infections (e.g. orthopaedic devices). When micro-organisms have adhered to a biomaterial surface they are protected against phagocytosis, as the micro-organism and biomaterial together are too large to ingest. Zimmerli *et al.*[10] reported that the activity of phagocytosis and polymorphonuclear leukocytes is decreased in the presence of a biomaterial. Little, however, is known about biofilm formation on implanted surgical meshes in the abdominal wall. Common biofilm-forming bacterial species on sutures, which are made of similar materials to that of surgical meshes, are *S. aureus* and *S. epidermidis*. In vascular grafts, commonly made of ePTFE, these are mainly Gram-positive cocci. Enteric micro-organisms (e.g. *Escherichia coli* and enterococcal strains) are also known to be capable of biofilm formation, and thus have to be considered as relevant species for abdominal wall implant infections, especially when intra-abdominal surgical techniques and placement of the mesh are involved.

In several clinical studies, micro-organisms that have caused abdominal wall implant infection have been determined (see Table 2). *S. aureus*, *S. epidermidis* and *E. coli* reported as the cause of the mesh infection in the majority of cases. Almost all studies on abdominal wall implant infections report the presence of multiple bacterial strains per patient. Therefore, long-lasting infections on surgical meshes in the abdominal wall should be considered as consisting of multiple different bacterial strains. This yields that the options for treatment of these infections are narrowed due to strain-dependent action of antibiotic agents.

Biomaterials Properties Involved in Biofilm Formation

Little information is available about the dependence of bacterial adhesion on the actual chemical composition of polymeric surfaces. Speranza *et al.*[19] showed in an experimental study using *E. coli* that the Lewis acid-base interaction between surface and micro-organism plays an important role in strengthening bacterial adhesion. Gottenbos *et al.*[20] showed that positively charged disks decrease the growth potential of Gram-negative bacteria, such as *E. coli*, in a rat-model. On the other hand, negatively charged mesh biomaterials facilitate host cell adhesion, growth and proliferation and host vessel ingrowth, which will indirectly protect the biomaterial from colonization of micro-organisms. Furthermore, specific chemical surface interactions between micro-organism and biomaterial or its conditioning film strengthen or reduce adhesion.

Table 2.   An Overview of Reports on Isolated Bacterial Strains from Abdominal Wall Infections after Abdominal Wall Reconstructive Surgery with or without the Use of a Surgical Mesh

Author	Mesh Material	Surgical Indication	Isolated Bacterial Strain
Rios *et al.*[11]	PP	Incisional hernia repair	*S. aureus* *S. epidermidis* *Streptococcus pyogenes*
Petersen *et al.*[12]	PP	Incisional hernia repair	*S. aureus* *Coagulase negative Staphylococcus* *β-hemolytic streptococcus*
	ePTFE	Incisional hernia repair	*S. aureus* *E. coli* *Enterococcus* *Coagulase negative Staphylococcus*
	POL	Incisional hernia repair	*Coagulase negative Staphylococcus* *Acinetobacter baumanii*
Miranda *et al.*[13]	No mesh	Hysterectomy	*S. aureus* *Mycoplasma hominis* *E. coli*
Taylor and O'Dweyer[14]	Not reported	Inguinal hernia repair	*S. aureus* *Proteus* *Group B streptococcal strains* *Peptostreptococci*
Case reports[15-18]	PP, ePTFE	Ventral and inguinal hernia repair	*Mycobacterium fortuitum* *Staphylococcus lugdunensis* *Mycobactrerium goodie* *Methicilin-resistant S. aureus*

Wettability depends either on the material of which the surface consists or on the conditioning film on the substratum surface. For example, metal surfaces are hydrophilic, as shown by low water contact angles, and are negatively charged. Polymers, such as PP or PTFE, are hydrophobic, as shown by high water contact angles, and are less electrostatically charged (see Table 1 for water contact angles). Bacterial adherence on surfaces is influenced by the wettability of the material, bacterial strain and material type. Decreased wettability, with lower water contact angles, reduces the incidence of attachment of *E. coli* during the reversible first phase of bacterial adhesion on the biomaterial surface. *S. aureus* has shown significantly less adhesive potential to extremely hydrophobic ePTFE patches compared to less hydrophobic PP mesh. As shown in the next paragraph, wettability directly influences protein adsorption on the biomaterial surface, and thus the composition of the conditioning film surrounding the biomaterial. The composition of the conditioning film influences host tissue ingrowth and bacterial adhesion and colonization on the biomaterial surface.

Environmental Properties and Conditioning Film

Adhesive potential and the formation of a biofilm on an implant device depends on the environment in which the device is introduced and the material aspects of the mesh itself. Proteins from the environment are adapted in a fluid-protein layer, the so-called conditioning film, surrounding the implanted device. This layer directly influences potential of adhesion and the potential of forming an infection threat of micro-organisms. In addition, physico-chemical material properties of the implant have shown to be of significant influence on the composition of the conditioning film. The characteristics of the conditioning film are of great influence on the type of biofilm that will grow on it.

In the abdominal wall, the mesh is surrounded with blood and interstitial fluid, in which proteins like albumin, immunoglobulin, fibrinogen and fibrinectin are present. Hydrophobic surfaces have a higher affinity for the adhesion of complement C3, fibronectin and vitronectin compared to a higher absorption of IgG and albumin on hydrophilic surfaces. In this regard, it is known that a hydrophobic surface, e.g. Marlex® and Gore-Tex® meshes, adsorbs less proteins with relatively more albumin, when exposed to blood serum. In contrast, with hydrophilic surfaces, e.g. Bard Teflon® and Fluoropassiv® meshes, a higher concentration of fibrinogen is found in the conditioning film.

Francois *et al.*[21] have described molecular mechanisms of *S. aureus* attachment to host protein-coated biomedical implants. These interactions involve specific surface proteins, so-called bacterial adhesins, which recognize specific domains of host proteins deposited as a film on indwelling devices, such as fibronectin, fibrinogen, fibrin or albumin. In addition, in a study with central venous catheters coated with plasma proteins, a major contribution to the adhesion and colonization of *S. aureus* was delivered by fibronectin and fibrinogen. Albumin is, for unclear reasons, a strong adhesion inhibitor, although changes in wettability and steric hindrance are proposed mechanisms.

Mono- and Multifilament Yarns

To create a strong mesh, the diameter of the threads can be made larger and formed into a monofilament mesh, or several threads can be woven or knitted together to form a dual- or multifilament mesh. Several studies have reported results on the effects of the number of filaments on bacterial colonization. In 1982, Sharp *et al.*[22] analyzed the effect of 16 different suture materials on the infection rate in mice. They found lower rates in monofilament materials in comparison to multifilament materials. In 1979, Österberg and Blomstedt[23] reported an increased inflammatory tissue reaction in the presence of *S. aureus* with multifilament sutures, in particular. Furthermore, they found a significantly increased persistence of bacteria in the wound for up to 41 days after surgery for multifilament sutures compared to monofilament sutures. Klinge *et al.*[2] showed in their study a significantly higher adherence rate of *S. aureus* in multifilament PP meshes compared to monofilament PP meshes. They concluded that the large surface area and the existence of niches in multifilament meshes promote the persistence of bacteria in the implant bed, by directly influencing the surface roughness and, secondarily, surface wettability (see paragraph 4.2). The data Merritt[24] has gathered, confirms that the infection rate with multifilament sutures (or porous materials) is greater than that with monofilament sutures (or solid materials) when the organisms are encountered at implantation (acute model) and indicate that a significant risk of infection may occur when only a few organisms are on a device at implantation. Even in highly sterilized alloplastic operations bacterial colonization has been observed in up to 40% of cases. Therefore, multifilament meshes are thought to increase the infection rate.

Multifilament yarns also induce a thicker and more compact collagen build-up, which could be a result of the stronger inflammatory reaction induced by the multifilament yarns compared to monofilament yarns. The thicker and more compacted collagen bundles are created around multifilament yarns, so the natural tensile strength of the surrounding tissue is probably higher.

Dual-filament meshes are available, but studies in which the infection rate is systematically compared to monofilament or multifilament materials have not been conducted. Multifilament materials are thought to be at significantly higher risk for bacterial colonization due to its increased surface area compared to monofilament yarns. The existence of niches prevents the host tissue ingrowth and inflammatory reaction from eradicating all bacteria. These bacteria are able to stay on the surface of the implanted material for years and produce late infections or abscess formation. Also, bacteria have the opportunity to form a biofilm and be counter-productive to the integration of the biomaterial. In hernia repair this can lead to insufficient adherence of host tissue and failure of the implant.

Prevention of Mesh Infection

A biofilm on a surface is capable of resisting antimicrobial agents due to the protective mechanisms expressed by the micro-organism. Once a biofilm has formed, it should be considered too late for initiation of antibiotic treatment, and the only option for treatment is now removal of the implanted device. Therefore, adequate prevention of a full-blown biomaterial-centered infection should aim at the first contact of a micro-organism with a biomaterial. Studies on the prevention of biofilm formation are mainly focusing on altering the surface of a biomaterial to inhibit bacterial attachment and on reducing the bacterial load by reducing, by the use of antibiotics, the number of planktonic bacteria on the implant side. A fast and close incorporation by host tissue lowers the chance for bacteria to adhere on the biomaterial surface, and thus reduces infection rates. The theory behind these findings is that when the device is incorporated easily by the host, the host tissue and the host immune system are brought close to the biomaterial surface, optimizing the protection of the device from micro-organisms. Furthermore, when biocompatibility is low a barrier of fibro-connective tissue prevents the host immune system from migrating to the biomaterial surface. Therefore, increasing biocompatibility is considered to be of enormous value for the prevention of biomaterial-related infections.

Mesh Coating

Since bacterial adhesion on the biomaterial depends on the surface aspects of a device, coatings have been a subject of research for a long time. Several types of coatings on surgical meshes have been studied with regard to their infection rate, host tissue ingrowth and intestinal adhesion formation (see Table 3).

Klinge and colleagues[25] coated a PP mesh with absorbable PG, which resulted in a significantly elevated tissue ingrowth rate. Sharp *et al.*[22] concluded in a large study on natural and synthetic suture materials that lubricating coatings on suture materials has no effect on infection rates. In contrast to smoothening the material surface, decreased wettability seems to have an effect on the attachment of bacteria; polymers with a hydrophobic coating reduced the incidence of attachment of *E. coli*. Growth of Gram-negative bacteria is also reduced on polymers with a positively charged coating.

Several studies show that titanium coatings on PP lead to better biocompatibility and also reduce attachment of micro-organisms. W. L. Gore & Associates introduced an ePTFE mesh coated with two antimicrobial agents (silver carbonate and chlorhexidine diacetate), which inhibit bacterial colonization on the patch for up to 10 days post-implantation. More recently, gold and gold-palladium, which are both known as antimicrobial agents, were successfully coated on a PP mesh. Also, antimicrobial aspects of a silver coating were tested on a polyethylene terephthalate fabric,

Table 3.   A List of Biomaterials Coatings Used in Experimental Studies on Different Surgical Meshes for Abdominal Wall Reconstructions, with their Specific Actions on Host Tissue Ingrowth or Bacterial Colonization on the Material Surface

Research	Coating	Mesh Material	Action
Klinge et al.[25]	Polyglactin	PP	Increases host tissue ingrowth
Soares et al.[3]	Gelatin and fluorocarbon	POL	Increases biocompatibility
Lehle et al.[26,27] Scheidbach et al.[28] Junge et al.[29]	Titanium-carboxonitride	PP, PTFE	Increases host tissue ingrowth and reduces bacterial attachment
Saygun et al.[30]	Gold, Gold-Palladium	PP	Prevents bacterial colonization
Klueh et al.[31]	Silver	Poly(ethylene) terephthalate fabric	Reduces bacterial attachment
Yelimlies et al.[32]	Carboxymethyl-cellulose	PP	Reduces the incidence of adhesions
Kapischke et al.[33] Kyzer et al.[34]	Human fibroblasts	PP, PGA	Yields positive effects on wound healing
Van 't Riet et al.[35]	Collagen	PP	Decreases adhesion formation, but increases infection rates
Sobinsky et al.[36]	Glucosaminoglycan-keratin luminal	PTFE	Initiates bacterial destruction

which successfully reduced bacterial attachment. In addition to research aimed at the antimicrobial functions of metals, some biochemical coatings have been tested in experimental studies. In these studies, carboxymethylcellulose coating (the combination of gelatin and fluorocarbon) together with PP, which was coated with human fibroblasts, did increase biocompatibility successfully. These findings are of great importance since the crucial strategy of preventing biomaterial-related infections is to prevent initial bacterial attachment and growth.

Antibiotics

As mentioned previously, bacterial susceptibility for a pharmacological treatment is significantly reduced when a polymeric devices is present. Prior to almost all procedures involving the implantation of a prosthetic device, antibiotics are administered with the aim to prevent peri-operative attachment of bacteria, although results from large double-blind studies suggest that the effect of this treatment is not confirmed. To be able to deliver antibiotics close to the biomaterial and additionally kill potentially adhesive micro-organisms, antimicrobial coatings have been developed. In an experimental study with dogs, cefoxitin-coated vascular PTFE grafts showed significant protection of the graft lumen during an induced bacteraemia. Despite these developments, clinical routine still uses a single prophylactic dose of systemic antibiotics at the moment of implantation to prevent biomaterial-centered infections in the recovering patient.

Recent Developments

Until recently, efforts to reduce infection have placed much emphasis on preventing bacterial colonization on biomaterials during the initial bacterial attachment stage, in addition to the changing policy on antibiotic prophylaxis. New insights have been reported on enzymatic interactions with biofilm formation. In a dental study, Kaplan and Ragunath[37] demonstrated the possibilities of enzymatic detachment of biofilms from synthetic surfaces. When a biofilm is detached it is more likely to be overtaken and cleared by antibiotics in combination with the host immune response. After positive results of human fibroblast-coated PGA meshes on wound healing,[34] Kapischke and colleagues[33] proved the feasibility of coating synthetic meshes with human fibroblasts. Nevertheless, both studies need further refinement in order to show the effects of the coatings on adhesion formation and clinical infection rates.

Several recent studies have looked into the effects of ultrasound on bacterial cell growth and their use in the treatment of biomaterial-centered infections. Ultrasound, however, cannot replace antibiotic treatment, since it reduces biofilm formation only selectively or, when applied in a too low-intensity, will even increase bacterial growth. The antimicrobial effect of antibiotics is enhanced when ultrasound is added to either systemic or locally applied (i.e. by means of a coating) antibiotic treatment. This phenomenon, based on the theory that ultrasound waves enhance the transportation and penetration of molecules in the biofilm, is called the bio-acoustic effect. In theory, this might result in higher nutrient concentrations in the biofilm, allowing it to grow faster. Also, when antibiotics are applied the penetration in the biofilm is enhanced, increasing the effect of the treatment. Several studies have shown ultrasound to have a positive effect when combined with gentamicin treatment against *E. coli*, and vancomycin treatment against *S. epidermidis*. With the contribution of low-frequency and high-intensity ultrasound in the presence of an antibiotic agent, micro-organisms may be removed and killed, which could be of major importance for the treatment of biomaterial-centered infections in the future.

References

1. Ramirez OM, Ruas E, Dellon AL. (1990) "Components separation" method for closure of abdominal-wall defects: an anatomic and clinical study. *Plas Rec Surg* **86**(3):519–26.
2. Klinge U, Junge K, Spellerberg B, *et al.* (2002) Do multifilament alloplastic meshes increase the infection rate? Analysis of the polymeric surface, the bacteria adherence, and the *in vivo* consequences in a rat model. *J Biomed Mater Res* **63**(6):765–71.
3. Soares BM, King MW, Marois Y, *et al.* (1996) *In vitro* characterization of a fluoropassivated gelatin-impregnated polyester mesh for hernia repair. *J Biomed Mater Res* **32**(2):259–70.
4. Hutchinson RW, Chagnon M, Divilio LT. (2000) *Preclinical Abdominal Adhesion Studies with Proceed Surgical Mesh.* Johnson & Johnson.
5. Amid PK. (1997) Classification of biomaterials and their related complications in abdominal wall hernia surgery. *Hernia* **1**:15–21.
6. Zhukovsky V, Rovinskaya L, Vinokurova T, Zhukovskaya I. (2002) The development and manufacture of polymeric endoprosthetic meshes for the surgery of soft tissues. *AUTEX Res J* **2**(4):204–9.
7. Ansaloni L, Catena F, D'Alessandro L. (2003) Prospective randomized, double-blind, controlled trial comparing Lichtenstein's repair of inguinal hernia with

polypropylene mesh versus Surgisis gold soft tissue graft: preliminary results. *Acta Biomed Ateneo Parmese* 74(suppl 2):10–14.

8. Gristina AG, Naylor P, Myrvik QN. (1988) Infections from biomaterials and implants: a race for the surface. *Med Prog Tech* 14(3–4):205–24.

9. Scott NW, McCormack K, Graham P, *et al.* EHTC Open Mesh versus non-Mesh for groin hernia repair. *Cochrane Datab Syst Rev*, 3:Art. No. CD002197.

10. Zimmerli W, Waldvogel FA, Vaudaux P, Nydegger UE. (1982) Pathogenesis of foreign body infection: description and characteristics of an animal model. *J Infect Dis* 146(4):487–97.

11. Rios A, Rodriguez JM, Munitiz V, *et al.* (2001) Antibiotic prophylaxis in incisional hernia repair using a prosthesis. *Hernia*, 5(3):148–52.

12. Petersen S, Henke G, Freitag M, *et al.* (2001) Deep prosthesis infection in incisional hernia repair: predictive factors and clinical outcome. *Eur J Surg* 167:453–7.

13. Miranda C, Alados JC, Molina JM, *et al.* (1993) Posthysterectomy wound infection. A review. *Diag Microb Infect Dis* 17(1):41–4.

14. Taylor SG, O'Dwyer PJ. (1999) Chronic groin sepsis following tension-free inguinal hernioplasty. *Br J Surg* 86:562–5.

15. Matthews MR, Caruso DM, Tsujimura RB, *et al.* (1999) Ventral hernia synthetic mesh repair infected by *Mycobacterium fortuitum*. *Am Surg* 65(11):1035–7.

16. Sanchez P, Buezas V, Maestre JR. (2001) *Staphylococcus lugdunensis* infection: report of thirteen cases. *Enferm Infec Microb Clin* 19(10):475–8.

17. Sohail MR, Smilack JD. (2004) Hernia repair mesh associated *Mycobacterium goodii* infection. *J Clin Microbiol* 42(6):2858–60.

18. Kercher KW, Sing RF, Matthews BD, Henifold BT. (2002) Successful salvage of infected PTFE mesh after ventral hernia repair. *Ost/Wound Manag* 48(10):40.

19. Speranza G, Gottardi G, Pederzolli C, *et al.* (2004) Role of chemical interactions in bacterial adhesion to polymer surfaces. *Biomaterials* 25(11):2029–37.

20. Gottenbos B, Van der Mei HC, Klatter F, *et al.* (2003) Positively charged biomaterials exert antimicrobial effects on gram-negative bacilli in rats. *Biomaterials* 24(16):2707–10.

21. Francois P, Vaudaux P, Foster TJ, Lew DP. (1996) Host-bacteria interactions in foreign body infections. *Inf Contr Hosp Epidemiol* 17(8):514–20.

22. Sharp WV, Belden TA, King PH, Teague PC. (1982) Suture resistance to infection. *Surgery* 91(1):61–3.

23. Osterberg B, Blomstedt B. (1979) Effect of suture materials on bacterial survival in infected wounds. An experimental study. *Acta Chir Scan* 145(7):431–4.

24. Merritt K. (1999) Tissue colonization from implantable biomaterials with low numbers of bacteria. *J Biomed Mater Res* 44(3):261–5.

25. Klinge U, Klosterhalfen B, Muller M, *et al.* (1999) Influence of polyglactin-coating on functional and morphological parameters of polypropylene-mesh modifications for abdominal wall repair. *Biomaterials* 20(7):613–23.

26. Lehle K, Lohn S, Reinerth GG, *et al.* (2004) Cytological evaluation of the tissue-implant reaction associated with subcutaneous implantation of polymers coated with titaniumcarboxonitride *in vivo. Biomaterials* 25(24):5457–66.

27. Lehle K, Buttstaedt J, Birnbaum DE. (2003) Expression of adhesion molecules and cytokines *in vitro* by endothelial cells seeded on various polymer surfaces coated with titaniumcarboxonitride. *J Biomed Mater Res* 65(3):393–401.

28. Scheidbach H, Tannapfel A, Schmidt U, *et al.* (2004) Influence of titanium coating on the biocompatibility of a heavyweight polypropylene mesh. An animal experimental model. *Eur Surg Res* 36(5):313–7.

29. Junge K, Rosch R, Klinge U, *et al.* (2005) Titanium coating of a polypropylene mesh for hernia repair: effect on biocompatibility. *Hernia* 9(2):115–9.

30. Saygun O, Agalar C, Aydinuraz K, *et al.* (2005) Gold and gold-palladium coated polypropylene grafts in a *Staphylococcus epidermidis* wound infection model. *J Surg Res*, epub April 28.

31. Klueh U, Wagner V, Kelly S, *et al.* (2000) Efficacy of silver-coated fabric to prevent bacterial colonization and subsequent device-based biofilm formation. *J Biomed Mater Res* 53(6):621–31.

32. Yelimlies B, Alponat A, Cubukcu A, *et al.* (2003) Carboxymethylcellulose coated on visceral face of polypropylene mesh prevents adhesion without impairing wound healing in incisional hernia model in rats. *Hernia* 7(3):130–3.

33. Kapischke M, Prinz K, Tepel J, *et al.* (2005) Precoating of alloplastic materials with living human fibroblasts — a feasibility study. *Surg Endosc* 19(6):791–7.

34. Kyzer S, Kadouri A, Levi A, *et al.* (1997) Repair of fascia with polyglycolic acid mesh cultured with fibroblasts — experimental study. *Eur Surg Res* 29(2):84–92.

35. Van 't Riet M, Burger JWA, Bonthuis F, *et al.* (2004) Prevention of adhesion formation to polypropylene mesh by collagen coating: a randomized controlled study in a rat model of ventral hernia repair. *Surg Endosc* 18(4):681–5.

36. Sobinsky KR, Flanigan DP. (1986) Antibiotic binding to polytetrafluoroethylene via glucosaminoglycan-keratin luminal coating. *Surgery* 100(4):629–34.

37. Kaplan, JB, Ragunath C. (2004) Enzymatic detachment of *Staphylococcus epidermidis* biofilms. *Antimicrob Agents Chemother* 48(7):2633–6.

Index

www.ingramcontent.com/pod-product-compliance
Lightning Source LLC
Chambersburg PA
CBHW060347220326
41598CB00023B/2837